Famous Doctors
and
Famous Patients

Famous Doctors and Famous Patients

Lives in Jeopardy?

Dr. Diane Holloway Cheney

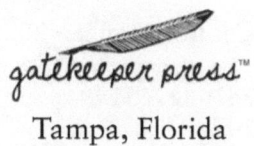

Tampa, Florida

The views and opinions expressed in this book are solely those of the author and do not reflect the views or opinions of Gatekeeper Press. Gatekeeper Press is not to be held responsible for and expressly disclaims responsibility for the content herein.

Famous Doctors and Famous Patients: Lives in Jeopardy?

Published by Gatekeeper Press
7853 Gunn Hwy., Suite 209
Tampa, FL 33626
www.GatekeeperPress.com

Copyright © 2024 by Dr. Diane Holloway Cheney
All rights reserved. Neither this book, nor any parts within it may be sold or reproduced in any form or by any electronic or mechanical means, including information storage and retrieval systems, without permission in writing from the author. The only exception is by a reviewer, who may quote short excerpts in a review.

Library of Congress Control Number: 2023947736

ISBN (paperback): 9781662945199
eISBN: 9781662945205

Table of Contents

Introduction vii

Chapter One   Sigmund Freud 1

Chapter Two   Max Schur, M.D. 8

Chapter Three Maynard Brandsma, M.D. 17
                Humphrey Bogart 28
                Ward Bond 36
                John Ford 38
                Rock Hudson 42
                Carole Landis 45
                Primula Niven (Mrs. David Niven) 49
                Dick Powell 53
                John Wayne 58

Chapter Four Ralph Greenson. M.D. 69
                Tony Curtis 74
                Celeste Holm 78
                Vivien Leigh 81
                Oscar Levant 85
                Peter Lorre 90
                Vincente Minelli 94
                Marilyn Monroe 98
                Frank Sinatra 105
                Inger Stevens 108

Chapter Five   Max Jacobson, M.D. 112
                Maria Callas 117
                Truman Capote 121
                Van Cliburn 125

	Rosemary Clooney 129
	Robert Cummings 132
	Cecile B. DeMille.................................... 139
	Marlene Dietrich.................................... 143
	Eddie Fisher 147
	John and Jacqueline Kennedy 150
	Hedy Lamarr 173
	Alan Jay Lerner....................................... 177
	Mickey Mantle 180
	Johnny Mathis.. 183
	Liza Minnelli 185
	Christopher Plummer............................. 188
	Anthony Quinn....................................... 191
	Edward G. Robinson 194
	Elizabeth Taylor..................................... 199
	Kay Thompson 202
	Billy Wilder..205
	Tennessee Williams................................209
Chapter Six	Timothy Leary, Ph.D. and Mortimer Hartman, M.D.................. 212
	Dan Aykroyd 217
	Johnny Depp... 219
	Betsy Drake 222
	Cary Grant 226
	Susan Sarandon 231
	Esther Williams 234
Chapter Seven	Menninger's Clinic 238
	Brett Favre.. 242
	Carl Panzram (American Serial Killer).....246
	Akim Tamiroff..252
	Gene Tierney 256
	Robert Walker 264
Chapter Eight	Selecting a Doctor 268

Introduction

During my life and work as a psychoanalytical psychologist, I and co-author, former rocket scientist, Edgar Van Cott, have met many famous doctors who are friends and colleagues.

We decided to lay out the lives of a few famous doctors and the lives of some of their famous patients. We will be examining what kind of doctor prescribed what kind of treatment. Nobody is perfect but most people presume that highly educated physicians will be helpful rather than harmful.

This seems particularly important with the statistics about "The Growing Gap in Life Expectancies Between the U.S. and Other Countries, 1933-2021." The United States has lower life expectancies than 56 countries, according to Steven H. Woolf, M.D., MPH. He published that article in 2023, *American Journal of Public Health,* 113 (9): pages 970-980. He listed the causes, and they include these factors: drugs, firearms, suicides, liver disease related to alcohol, diet and obesity, family disruptions, erosion in trust and social adherence, racism, and social media.

As we studied some seemingly good doctors, we found that some made their patients worse through treatments involving mind-altering drugs. I first became a nurse in the psychiatric unit of Parkland Hospital when President Kennedy and Lee Harvey Oswald died there. Next was training to be a psychologist for individuals and companies. I was later chosen by the mayor to be the Drug Czar for the

City of Dallas. Thus, much knowledge was gained about mind-altering chemicals that promise relief but impose problems upon the user. I obtained a three-million-dollar grant from the federal Office of Substance Abuse (OSAP) in 1987 for our Dallas Against Drugs program for which I was recognized at the White House under Ronald Reagan's U.S. Drug Czar William Bennett.

Co-author Ed Van Cott has experience in management. Managers accomplish tasks through others. Thus, a manager concentrates on goals, planning, and reporting progress to superiors. The secret is delegation of tasks to subordinates who report progress periodically. When tasks are successfully completed, those involved receive the satisfaction of accomplishment.

Life is an adventure with many challenges along the way for doctors and patients. Patients seek another opinion if the doctor's recommendation is not believed to be appropriate. Often, the patient has a better understanding of their body and how it feels than outsiders like doctors do.

Doctors are challenged to find better treatments for new diseases. They are also challenged to understand the patient's mental and emotional needs. Patients are challenged to find a doctor that can help them cure conditions that cause illness or stress. When successful, both the doctor and patient receive the satisfaction of accomplishment and hopefully, the patient improves.

Each person in this world tries to cope with various life difficulties, but we often ask the aid of physicians to help us with medical problems, relief of pain, stress, and good health. Since all doctors are also patients, we will proceed with Sigmund Freud, Maynard Brandsma,

Ralph Greenson, Max Jacobson, Timothy Leary, and Karl Menninger. Biographical information from *Wikipedia* was useful as well as other references cited.

The book will conclude with some thoughts about selecting good doctors.

CHAPTER ONE
Sigmund Freud

Sigmund Freud (1856 – 1939) was an Austrian neurologist who developed the field of psychoanalysis. He is considered one of the most influential thinkers of the Twentieth Century, even though many of his ideas have been challenged in recent decades.

Freud was born May 6, 1856, in Freiberg in Moravia, Austrian Empire (now Příbor, Czech Republic) to Hasidic Jewish parents. He was brought up in Leipzig and Vienna, and proved to be an outstanding student, excelling in languages and English literature. He developed a love for reading Shakespeare in original English. At the age of seventeen, Freud joined the medical faculty at the University of Vienna to study subjects such as philosophy, physiology, and zoology.

Freud graduated in 1881 and began working at the Vienna General Hospital. He worked in various departments, such as the psychiatric clinic and combined medical practice with research with an 1891 paper on aphasia (the inability to express or understand spoken language) and 1894 paper on the effects of cocaine. Freud was initially an advocate of using cocaine for pain relief, though he later reconsidered as its dangers became increasingly known.

While working in different medical fields, Freud continued his own independent reading. He was influenced by Charles Darwin's relatively new theory of evolution. Sigmund read Friedrich Nietzsche's philosophy extensively. He also studied the practice of hypnosis, as developed by Jean-Martin Charcot in Paris.

In 1886, Freud left his hospital post and set up a private clinic specializing in nervous disorders. An important aspect of Freud's approach was to encourage patients to share their innermost thoughts and feelings, which often lay buried in their subconscious. Initially, he used hypnosis, but later found he could just ask people to talk about their past and their experiences.

He realized that listening may be the sincerest form of flattery and made patients want to talk about themselves. Dale Carnegie (1888-1955) wrote *How to Win Friends and Influence People* in 1937. He wrote, "You can make more friends in two weeks by becoming a good listener than you can in two years trying to get other people interested in you."

What is a good listener? They look at the speaker, do not interrupt, focus on understanding, suspend judgment, sum up at intervals, ask questions to clarify, determine the need at the moment, and keep their emotions under control while listening. Freud eventually changed from looking directly at patients to sitting behind them, so his face and body movements did not make people feel judged. Listening allows people to feel they are approved of and are deemed a good person.

President Harry Truman said something along that line. "When we understand the other fellow's viewpoint, nine times out of ten, he is trying to do right." Listening suggests that a person is acceptable. Even President Abraham Lincoln described the need for self-acceptance. He said,

"When I lay down the reins of this administration, I want to have one friend left. And that friend is inside myself."

Freud began to realize that we are first influenced by what we see our parents doing. Parents mean to mentor their children and pass on what they have learned. However, sometimes they behave in a bad manner that causes their child to copy that unruly behavior. On the other hand, people sometimes feel rather fond or romantic about their parents. Hence, the old song "I want a girl, just like the girl that married dear old dad." For girls, the Gershwin song "Someone to Watch Over Me" suggested that a girl thinks of a boyfriend like a father in the line "I know I'll always be good to someone who'll watch over me."

Freud hoped that by bringing the unconscious thoughts and feelings to the surface, patients would be able to let go of repetitive negative emotions and feelings. Another technique he pioneered was 'transference' which showed patients how they would often transfer feelings about others onto the psychoanalyst, whose background they knew little about. For example, if a female had a father who was unfaithful, she might expect all men to be unfaithful, and she might imagine that her analyst was trying to seduce her. The Hippocratic oath and rules of each health profession forbid personal relationships between patients and doctors. That practice reduces the chance that a professional would take advantage of a personal relationship to benefit themselves outside of their fee for service.

In 1899, Freud published *'The Interpretation of Dreams'* in which he suggested that dreams are often about unfulfilled wishes. We dream about what we are struggling with, as if we are trying or practicing how to solve a problem in the dream. He later applied his theories to daily life, which generated a larger readership among the public. Such works were *The Psychopathology of Everyday Life* (1901), *Jokes and their Relation to the Unconscious* (1905), and *Three Essays on the Theory of Sexuality* (1905).

From the early 1900s, Freud's new theories became increasingly influential – attracting followers interested in the new theories of psychology. Other notable members of his group included Jews such as Wilhelm Stekel, Alfred Adler, Max Kahane, and Rudolf Reitler. The group discussed ideas about the mind, and by 1908, this group had become larger and was formalized as the Vienna Psychoanalytic Society. The subdued voices were speaking most of the principle European tongues.

In 1909 and 1910, Freud's ideas were increasingly spread to the English-speaking world. With Carl Jung, Freud visited New York in 1909. The trip was a success with Freud awarded an Honorary Doctorate from Clark University in Massachusetts. This led to considerable media interest and the later formation of the American Psychoanalytic Association in 1911. However, as the movement grew, there were increasing philosophical splits, with key members taking different approaches. However, Freud and the field of psychoanalysis continued to grow in prominence.

In 1930, Sigmund Freud was awarded the Goethe Prize for his contributions to German literature and psychology. Johann Wolfgang von Goethe had said, "Treat a man as if he already were what he potentially could be, and you make him what he should be." Goethe believed that most people would do anything to live up to your faith in them.

After the mid-1920s, Freud also increasingly began to apply his theories to other fields such as history, art, literature, and anthropology. In 1925, the movie mogul

Samuel Goldwyn called Sigmund Freud the "greatest love specialist in the world." Goldwyn traveled all the way to Vienna to meet Sigmund Freud. He wanted to offer Freud $100,000 to collaborate on a film love story about Anthony and Cleopatra. Goldwyn wanted the famous doctor to tell filmmakers what was really happening in famous love stories. Freud, however, refused to see Goldwyn.[1]

The psychoanalyst summarized his feelings in a letter to a friend, saying, "Filming seems to be as unavoidable as page-boy haircuts, but I won't have myself trimmed that way and do not wish to be brought into personal contact with any film."

Freud did write a letter to a friend about Charlie Chaplin's movies. The works of all artists, claimed Freud, are "intimately bound up with their childhood memories," and Chaplin was no exception. Freud had seen some Chaplin films and here is a bit of that letter:

> You know for instance, in the last few days Charlie Chaplin has been in Vienna. I, too, would have seen him, but it was too cold for him here and he left again quickly. He is undoubtedly a great artist; certainly, he always portrays one and the same figure; only the weak, poor, helpless, clumsy youngster for whom, however, things turn out well in the end. Now do you think that for this role he has to forget his own ego? On the contrary, he always plays only himself as he was in his early dismal youth. He cannot get away from those impressions and to this day he obtains for himself compensation for the frustrations and humiliations of that past period of his life. He is, so-to-speak, an exceptionally simple and transparent

case. The idea that the achievements of artists are intimately bound up with their childhood memories, impressions, repressions, and disappointments, has already brought us much enlightenment.[2]

In 1933, the Nazi's came to power in Germany, and Freud's works as a Jewish writer were put on the list of prohibited books. Freud wryly remarked that we were making progress because in the Middle Ages they would have burned him, but now they were content with burning his books.

In 1938, Hitler secured an Anschluss of Germany and Austria which placed all Jewish people in great peril, especially intellectuals. In March 1938, daughter Anna Freud was detained by the Gestapo and Sigmund became more aware of how dire the situation was. With the help of Welsh psychoanalyst Ernest Jones (then president of the International Psychoanalytic Association), Freud and seventeen colleagues were given work permits to emigrate to Britain. Freud needed the help of sympathetic colleagues and friends to hide bank accounts and gain the necessary funds for travel to the United Kingdom.

When leaving Austria, Freud was required to sign a document testifying that he had been fairly treated. He did so, with a dry wit, adding in his own hand: *"I can most highly recommend the Gestapo to everyone."*[3]

Freud finally managed to leave Austria on June 4, 1938, by the Orient Express arriving in London on June 6. For the rest of his life, Freud lived at Hampstead, England, where he continued to write and see a few patients.

In 1923, Freud had been diagnosed with cancer from smoking cigars. The surgery on his jaw was partially successful, but by 1939, the cancer of his jaw got progressively worse, putting him in great pain. He died on 23 September 1939.

Freud was instrumental in the growth of psychoanalysis. He felt it to be his task on earth to call things by their right name and to illuminate the unconscious. His theories and writings have proved controversial but have often served as reference points for those who do talking therapy like psychologists, psychiatrists, social workers, etc.[4]

Let us now observe the relationship between Dr. Sigmund Freud and his physician Dr. Max Schur.

Notes

1. "When Hollywood's Elite Became Obsessed with Freudian Shrinks" by Matthew Sweet. https://www.thetimes.co.uk/article/when-hollywoods-elite-became-obsessed-with-freudianshrinks-75khdc6ks
2. https://www.mentalfloss.com/article/67137/time-sigmund-freud-analyzed-charlie-chaplin
3. http://www.prospectmagazine.co.uk/features/freud-the-last-great-enlightenment-thinker/
4. Pettinger, Tejvan. "Biography Sigmund Freud," Oxford, www.biographyonline.net, 23 March 2015.

CHAPTER TWO
Max Schur, M.D.

Dr. Max Schur (1897-1969) was a physician and friend of Freud who assisted him in euthanasia at the end of his life. Max was a Jew, attended medical school at the University of Vienna from 1915-1920, and attended Freud's *Introductory Lectures.* He had a personal analysis and was accepted in the Vienna Psychoanalytic Society in 1932. He became Freud's physician in 1929. At their initial meeting about his health, Freud asked Schur, "Promise me also when the time comes, you won't let them torment me unnecessarily." Ten years later in 1939, Freud approached death from cancer and Freud reminded him of that promise. Schur assured Freud that he would give him adequate sedation to end his life of pain.

Max Schur's son, Peter Schur, attended Harvard Medical School and contributed this description of Freud's death at the hands of his father. This description has now been gratefully received by so many who have studied Freud's life and are profoundly grateful for this information about the end of this unique man's life.[1]

This article is available for all to read in the autumn issue of 2013 *Harvard Medicine: The Magazine of Harvard Medical School.* It is entitled "Three Coins from Freud: A doctor-patient relationship spans nations and generations" by Peter Schur. Dr. Schur described Freud having fired another physician who tried to keep the truth about his fatal cancer from the psychoanalyst. That is why Freud sought out another physician who would be truthful with him about everything.

There are many reasons why physicians do not give patients news of a terminal diagnosis. They only have so much time and patients would naturally want to question things they are told. Doctors sometimes have rather distant long-term doctor-patient relationships, especially when they are terribly busy. Physicians hate to admit defeat or a lack of effective therapies to treat a disease. There is also a simple lack of physician communication, which is now being taught more carefully in medical schools. Patients have a right to their own data, including negative findings, and physicians must remain focused on the patient in these matters.

Here is the article about Dr. Schur's treatment of Dr. Sigmund Freud.

On May 6, 1933, my father, Max Schur, was examining Sigmund Freud. By this time, my father had served as Freud's physician for four years, overseeing his general care—Freud suffered from a heart condition—but especially monitoring and treating the oral lesions that plagued Freud.

My father had become Freud's physician after being recommended by Marie Bonaparte, the French author and psychoanalyst who was the great grandniece of Napoleon. Bonaparte had been in Vienna undergoing psychoanalysis with Freud and had need of an internal medicine physician. Coincidentally, Freud had fired his personal physician after learning that the man had kept from him the truth about the malignancy of his oral lesions. Thus, my father began a doctor–patient relationship that endured for 10 years, a decade that would turn out to be a tumultuous one worldwide.

On that day in May, however, Freud was marking his 77th birthday, and my father was awaiting the birth of his first child: me. My mother, Helen, herself a physician, was overdue, a fact that I'm told led Freud to urge my father to go to her side, saying, "You are going from a man who doesn't want to leave this world to a child who doesn't want to come into it." Three days later, I was born. In honor of my birth, Freud gave me three Austrian gold coins.

Remarkably, I still have those coins. I've kept one. The others I've distributed to my two daughters, so that they each may have something to remind them of the Schur–Freud connection that, in its small way, helped shape history.

The world I came into, Vienna in 1933, was a world in turmoil. The day following my birth, for example, the newspapers reported the burning of Freud's works, an act justified as one "against the soul-destroying overestimation of the sex life—and on behalf of the nobility of the human soul." The birth of their son, Peter, brought joy to Max and Helen Schur at a time when much of their world was poised for sorrow.

In March of that year, neighboring Germany had placed Hitler in power and Nazism was on the rise. With that menace so near, many members of the Jewish population were fleeing, including Freud's sons and their families. Austria, weakened by a civil war incited by Nazi coalitions within the country, was allying itself with Italy's Benito Mussolini. In the unsettled period following the assassination of Austria's Chancellor Engelbert Dollfus, friends and family urged Freud and my father to leave. My father had gone so far as to apply for positions outside Austria, including one in Cairo. But Freud could not be persuaded, and my father, in deference to his patient, stayed. So did we.

In February 1938, Hitler handed Dollfus's successor, Kurt von Schuschnigg, an ultimatum: capitulate or be invaded. While Schuschnigg considered Austria's options, my father went to the U.S. embassy to follow up on a visa application he had made the previous year under the Polish quota. My father had been born in 1897 in Stanislaw, a city that was then part of the Austro-Hungarian Empire, but which had, in 1919, become part of Poland: thus, he was considered Polish. My father also urged Freud to leave. Freud refused. Soon it was too late for everyone: The German army invaded Austria on March 12 and annexed the country. The *Anschluss* had taken place.

The next few weeks were tense. My parents continued to go to work at the hospital and kindergarten. Many of our neighbors flew Nazi flags. There were parades. I remember my parents being afraid. In particular, I remember an episode when Nazis came to our house. I was on the steps leading upstairs. My father was asked about his possessions, and gave over his automobile; an unloaded, fancy revolver; and some gold coins. I was very upset about losing the car, for I remembered riding in it with my father during many pleasurable trips taken around Vienna.

As frightening as that visit was, my parents were thankful that nothing worse had happened. They knew of the concentration camps and exterminations in Germany. Their efforts to leave the country intensified. Soon, through the political connections of many, including Paris-based Marie Bonaparte, exit visas and permit papers for the Freuds, my family, and others were procured.

On June 4, we were about to leave for London with the Freuds when my father developed acute severe phlegmonous appendicitis. The Freuds left, but we stayed while my father underwent an emergency appendectomy performed by an "Aryan" surgeon: At that time, few Jewish patients were admitted to hospitals and no Jewish physicians were allowed to practice in the hospitals. The Gestapo monitored my father closely; there were interactions between them and my father and mother at the hospital, at our home, and at Gestapo headquarters. Eventually, on June 10, we were allowed to leave. I remember my father arriving at the train station in a wheelchair, still bandaged, with a drain in his abdomen. The next day we arrived in Paris. We stayed there for three days while my father convalesced, then we traveled to London to join the Freuds.

In London, the routine between my father and Freud resumed. But Freud's malignant oral lesions recurred, and, in February 1939, a lesion developed that was deemed inoperable. After consultations, radiation therapy was begun.

Freud's end is well known and has been detailed by many. Early in their association, Freud had exacted a promise from my father that he would not allow Freud to die a tortured death. Freud now reminded my father of that conversation and asked him to fulfill his promise. My father consulted with Freud's daughter, Anna, and, on September 21, 1939, when Freud was again in agony, administered a one-third grain of morphine. His pain relieved, Freud fell into a peaceful sleep, then lapsed into a coma and died at 3 a.m. on September 23.

With Freud's death, my father's obligations to his patient were fulfilled, and we could join the masses of people fleeing Europe. In October, we obtained passage on the *SS President Harding*, sailing from Southampton, England, and stopping in France for additional passengers on its way to the United States. I slept on a cot in the ship's former drawing room with others, including my mother and my sister, Eva. My six-year-old self remembers our picking up survivors drifting in lifeboats following an attack by a German U-boat, and watching as British warships circled a burning vessel. I also remember that we were hit by a hurricane. From news reports I now know that one crew member died in that storm of October 17, and that 73 passengers and crew were injured, some severely. But I remember that right before the brunt of the storm hit, my mother performed an emergency appendectomy on one of the crew, with my father administering anesthesia, and the ship's doctor, fresh out of medical school, assisting.

When a tidal wave from the hurricane hit, I ended up under a pile of broken cots, unscathed. I stayed in a corridor for a few hours wearing a life preserver as water occasionally swished around, and protecting Eva, as my parents attended to more than 100 fractures. The next night we all slept in one bed in a cabin. The next day a U.S. warship passed medical supplies to the ship via a line. In New York City, we moved first to the Hotel Anderson, at 80th Street and Columbus Avenue, then to 515 West End Avenue. I attended PS9.

My father resumed his private practice of internal medicine. He applied for hospital privileges and was told by all, except Bellevue Hospital, that they did not accept refugees or Jews. At Bellevue he became an internist in the Division of Syphilology and Dermatology. He renewed his interest in analysis and became a member of the British and New York psychoanalytic associations, eventually cofounding the Psychoanalytic Association of New York (Downstate).

In the late 1950s, he gave up internal medicine to practice analysis full time. He quit Bellevue and joined the Department of Psychiatry, Downstate NY Medical Center in Brooklyn, where he eventually became a clinical professor. In the late 1960s, he was president of the American Psychoanalytic Association.

My mother became affiliated with the Department of Orthopedics at Mt. Sinai Hospital in New York, where she eventually ran the polio unit, including the respirators, as well as the posture clinic, in the days before rehabilitation units. When vaccines vanquished polio, my mother switched careers and took a five-year residency in adult, child, and adolescent psychiatry at Downstate. This was followed by training in childhood and adolescent analysis. Before being required to retire by New York State (at age 85), she was an assistant professor of psychiatry. Until shortly before her death, my mother continued to see private patients and to work in a children's clinic in East Harlem.

In the fall of 1969, my father contracted the flu and possibly developed pneumonia. On October 12 of that year, he died in his sleep. My mother outlived him, and collaborator to the end, wrote the preface to his book, *Freud: Living and Dying,* published in 1972.

The Schur–Freud connection lingers on in me. After graduating from elementary school, I attended Fieldston High School and went on to attend Yale College. In 1954, I entered Harvard Medical School, graduating in 1958. Anna Freud provided both Yale and HMS with wonderful, strong letters supporting my applications. During the years my father had cared for Freud, I had met Anna on several occasions. I recall her as a small, kind, fragile-looking lady.

In 1967, I joined the faculty at Harvard Medical School, and, in 1978, became a professor of medicine at what is now Brigham and Women's Hospital. My clinical and research interests have focused on systemic lupus erythematosus. I have, over the years, become interested in the psychopathology of that disease and of illness in general. This, I suppose, is another way in which the Schur–Freud connection endures.

Much has been written about this connection, and I have often been asked, "What about the connection hasn't been told?" I can add nothing, for my father, as Freud's physician, was discreet about what could be said. If he felt something could not be said, he mentioned it to no one, neither my mother, myself, nor others. I understand that. I feel that is the type of respect that all physicians owe to their patients. I am my father's son.

(Peter Schur '58 is an HMS professor of medicine in the Department of Rheumatology and Immunology at Brigham and Women's Hospital.)

Note

1. https://magazine.hms.harvard.edu/articles/three-coins-freud

CHAPTER THREE
Maynard Brandsma, M.D.

Dr. Maynard Grant Brandsma (1907-1999) was born in Holland and died in Mission Viejo, California. Co-author Edgar Van Cott worked for many years at Raytheon in Massachusetts as a rocket scientist. Then Ed, his wife, and mother moved in 1978 to Mission Viejo, California, to accept a position as president of a small company in Santa Ana, California. He purchased a house on Amapola Lane in Mission Viejo overlooking the Mission Viejo Golf Course. The area was known as "Pill Hill" due to many doctors in residence.

The house next door was owned by Dr. Maynard Brandsma whose wife, Mickie, was a realtor. She was of immense help to those new to the area. Soon Maynard, Mickie, Betty, and Ed became frequent dinner companions. As the wives prepared gourmet meals, Maynard would describe many of his adventures to Ed. The subject would vary with each dinner over several years.

Maynard remembered that his father was often away, and he was brought up more by his grandfather who encouraged him in the field of medicine. The grandfather had a highly active business and social life as he was successfully sued for child support at the age of 88 but died at 90 from slipping on ice.

One of Maynard's summer jobs was working in a cognac or brandy brewery. He remembered it was easy to get tipsy after breathing the fumes for only half a day. Maynard mentioned rowing as a sport. Two Brandsma's rowed in the 1924 Olympics when Maynard was seventeen. At age 17, Brandsma entered the Amsterdam Medical School. Following an internship, he served his residency under Dr. I Snapper, a renowned physician whom he termed "a tough man who was a walking medical encyclopedia."

Having learned much about medicine but little about the world, he began to lust for strange countries and fresh sights. Dr. Brandsma decided to become a ship's doctor and in 1933 began traveling throughout the continents. He settled down on a plantation in New Guinea for nearly a year and saw poverty, disease and a few native tribes still involved in head shrinking.

Dr. Brandsma left New Guinea and spent time traveling through Indonesia. Maynard also served as a fighter pilot in the Dutch Air Force in Indonesia. He eventually settled for a period in Batavia which is now called Djakarta. He described the clinic's doctor as an alcoholic for whom he had to take over as chief.

The Dutch East Indies (c. 1600–1942) was part of a vast Dutch trading empire which stretched across the world. In the 1400-1600s, the Spanish, (including Columbus), Portuguese, Arab, English, and Dutch traders were all keen to exploit the natural resources of islands in the south-east Asian archipelago and the 'New World' of the Americas. Nutmeg and cloves were highly sought in Europe as medicines and food. They were also thought to ward off the plague and thus were regarded as extremely valuable in social and economic terms. Most of these spices – including cinnamon and mace – grew only on a handful of islands and had been traded for hundreds of years.

The clinic included a house with servants and a garden. A boa constrictor was kept in the garden to eliminate rats and other vermin. When a new person was hired to work at the house, they were introduced to the boa so their scent would be recognized. Thus, like a dog recognizing scents, it would not attack a newcomer.

One medical incident occurred and Dr. Brandsma was called to a native village for sickness. After surveying the situation, the village chief was told by Dr. Brandsma to move the village a mile upstream and burn down the current village to destroy the disease. The village chief showed his appreciation by making two of his daughters available for the night. After that evening, Maynard returned to the clinic and drank a bottle of Dutch gin as medication. Gin and tonic containing quinine were used for malaria and venereal disease in those days. Winston Churchill once declared: "A gin and tonic has saved more Englishmen's lives and minds than all the doctors in the Empire."

Apparently, gin and tonic could not cure everything. Dr. Brandsma became terribly ill in Djakarta, and he began losing a great deal of weight. His friends convinced him to move to the United States and where he could convey his experiences to others through teaching. References from Netherlands physicians for contacts in California helped him find employment, as he had not taken or passed U.S. medical exams to become a licensed physician there. One contact identified a job teaching at Yale University in New Haven, Connecticut.

Maynard arrived there in time for the massive 1938 hurricane. This was before hurricanes received their names. Southern Connecticut news highlights noted that the hurricane made a landfall between Bridgeport and New Haven as a Category 3 and a 115-mph sustained wind. Hundreds of lives were lost with many injured. There was extensive damage to homes, trees, crops, bridges, utilities, and railroads were wiped out. There was also catastrophic damage to fishing fleets. Dr. Brandsma's medical expertise was extremely valuable at that time.

After a brief time in Connecticut, he accepted a teaching position at Stanford University in California and was consulted about his expertise in tropical diseases since the Defense department anticipated a conflict in the Pacific Ocean. Brains are like hearts—they go where they are appreciated. But that position did not last long for someone so experienced and talented.

In September 1939, President Roosevelt, a former assistant Secretary of the Navy under President Woodrow Wilson, suggested a confidential exchange of information to British First Lord of the Admiralty Winston Churchill. The Netherlands was invaded by Germany in 1940. In June 1940, William Stevenson went to New York to set up British Security Coordination based in Rockefeller Center which reported to the Prime Minister of Great Britain and the President of the United States.

In July 1941, Roosevelt appointed William Donovan to be chief of a centralized intelligence agency with the title of Coordinator of Information which evolved into the OSS (Office of Strategic Services). Stephenson and Donovan had known each other where they served in WWI.

By the outbreak of the second World War, Dr. Brandsma was teaching tropical medicine at the University of Southern California.

Soon after the war started, Dr. Brandsma joined the British Intelligence Force, a daring organization said to have only a 20 percent survival rate at that time. He reported under William Stephenson, the Canadian of "A Man called Intrepid' fame. The British saw the opportunity of enlisting a well-traveled and experienced physician, fluent in his native Dutch, French, German, English, Spanish and Malay.

Maynard told Ed about his 22-night parachute jumps into Europe, including one with William Stephenson. Before one jump, a crew chief pointed out a crew member that was the only survivor to return after several jumps. During the jump Maynard saw him signaling the ground with a flashlight. It became the saboteur's last jump because Maynard killed the traitor.

In June 1940, a new volunteer force called the Special Operations Executive (SOE) was set up to wage a secret war. Its agents were mainly tasked with sabotage and subversion behind enemy lines. Prime Minister Churchill ordered them to "Set Europe ablaze!" On a jump into Germany, he found himself behind enemy lines working as a waiter in a restaurant that was serving Hitler. Brandsma knew the poor fellow who was their behind the lines radio operator at the SOE and was eventually caught by the Nazi SS.

William Stephenson had identified Nork Hydro as the source of heavy water for German atomic experiments in October 1939. In 1940, he informed Churchill of a top-secret report that an atomic bomb could be constructed with heavy water. Maynard described a jump into Norway to destroy the heavily guarded Deuterium heavy water (D_2O) hydroelectric facility used to process uranium in Germany. Here is more about that attack.

Close to Oslo, Norway, there was a plant producing heavy water critical to the bomb project and shipping it to a laboratory in northern Germany. The plant was an enormous, impenetrable steel and concrete structure which had defied all attempts to destroy it, including seven 500-pound bombs dropped by the 8th Air Force. In a desperate attempt to wipe out the plant, 350 people were sent to Norway and only 26 survived. Brandsma knew five of them well and described them as reliable, effective agents. For his assigned project, he asked for volunteers, cautioning that the odds were against their survival. Three volunteered and he selected the two he knew best to go with him.

The three men entered the plant through an underwater sewer pipe in the cellar during the bitter cold of the Norwegian winter. Each man carried a load of TNT. Brandsma went to the top floor and directed the others to intervening levels. They placed their TNT in strategic spots. Miraculously, they met at the appointed site without being detected and made their way back to the safety of their hide-out. They met the other groups, picked up their gear, and began their ascent up the mountain when they heard the explosion. Turning, hoping to see complete destruction, Brandsma instead saw the plant still intact.

In total despair, they radioed headquarters. "Tried but failed." They waited tensely for nearly six hours and then word finally came that the interior of the plant had been destroyed. The order came: "Get the hell out. Go in small groups and don't get caught." The attack occurred on February 27 and 28 of 1943.

They knew that once before; an explosion had detonated inside the plant, but it was back in operation two days later. How could they be sure? The radio confirmed that the destruction was complete but a large shipment of heavy water in box cars to be ferried along the sound had escaped. Two Norwegians volunteered to place a timed charge on the ferry, set to go off when the boat was in water 2,000 feet deep. There were innocent people on board as well as the box cars but if heavy water were to reach its destination, Hitler would have his bomb. The charge exploded and the ferry sank to the bottom of the fjord. Later, intelligence confirmed that the Germans might have completed the bomb if Brandsma's heroic mission had been only five days later.

This was only one of twenty-eight missions undertaken by Maynard Brandsma in the service of his adopted country. Fortunately, and remarkably, he survived to tell the tale. The story of the attack on the plant in Norway where heavy water was being made for A-bombs was depicted in the 1965 movie *Heroes of Telemark* which starred Kirk Douglas, Richard Harris, and Michael Redgrave. The cellar at the site of the heavy water production company has recently been opened to the public.

Maynard said, "I would not have missed the experience of serving with the British, but memories become too severe and vivid to recall without some pain." He did not write about his war experiences because he found it too painful to dredge up those memories.

Maynard was called back into service during the Berlin Airlift crisis along with two dozen other pilots. They flew the airlift and identified and eliminated Russian saboteurs. Their reward was a one-week vacation in Paris with all expenses paid.

Many joined in the war effort after the attack on Pearl Harbor and declaration of war with Japan and Germany.

During the war, Maynard returned to California several times. There were plenty of women without escorts with many men overseas. In his single years, Maynard said he would not date a woman that had a husband in the service.

After the war ended, Maynard tended a bar in Las Vegas and developed a special martini (by adding a drop of Angostura bitter) while waiting for papers to clear him to open a medical practice in California. This drink increased his tip income as customers asked for his special martini. As an aside, he told Ed that he found Manhattan cocktails were best with Early Times Canadian Whiskey and sweet vermouth.

About this time, Maynard asked his own sober, weary heart if a new enthusiasm could still be in store for him. It was!

Dr. Brandsma started a clinic in Santa Monica around 1947 after receiving California medical credentials and treated movie stars such as Humphrey Bogart of 1942 *Casablanca* and the usual suspects including Ward Bond, John Ford, Greer Garson, Rock Hudson, Carole Landis, David Niven's wife Primmie, Dick Powell, and John Wayne and more. Some of the stars became his close companions and all had stories to tell, but few were as varied as Maynard's stories.

In an interesting aside, the head of Universal Studios who employed Rock Hudson, a former truck driver, called Maynard in one day and warned him about Hudson's big truck driver boyfriends. They asked Dr. Brandsma to keep Hudson's sexual orientation out of the papers, and he complied.

Maynard had a first wife who was Dutch, but nothing is known about that marriage except that his ex-wife married another man later in life. Ed met that very nice lady at Maynard's 90th birthday party.

Maynard married Roberta Grant in 1945 and they had three children. Maynard Jr. was born in 1947, became an engineer, and died in 2009 climbing Longs Peak at an elevation of 14,255 feet with his daughter. Kristin Honold was born 1949 and became a lawyer and retired to Albuquerque, New Mexico. Dana Black was born in 1950 and died in 2020 in Wickenburg, Arizona.

Dr. Brandsma was a member of the American College of Physicians by 1956 and served on several committees. They were living in Los Angeles in 1965 when his second wife Roberta died in a plane crash in 1965. Maynard had told her the pilot was not a good flyer and she should not fly with him. Maynard went to the crash site but would not allow his children to come along, which proved fortunate. He found parts of his wife's mangled body in a tree.

His son, Maynard Jr., was 17 years old, and the girls were 14 and 15. He wanted his teenagers to have a mother and sought a life partner that he could treasure. He chose Mildred "Mickie" Swanson who was born on June 11, 1925, on a farm near Big Sandy, Montana. She worked for the National Aeronautics and Space Administration in Los Angeles for many years. She also worked on the side as a medical records transcriber. While doing this work she met Maynard Brandsma who was so impressed with her that they were married in 1965 just a few months after his wife died.

In 1970, they moved to Mission Viejo where Ed Van Cott met them. After Mickie and Maynard settled in, she earned her real estate license. He first worked at Leisure World, a senior citizen community, but so many of his patients were dying that he left after a short time. He then started his own practice and contributed greatly to the founding and opening of the Mission Community Hospital in 1971. On the first weekend he personally admitted eighteen patients into the 124-bed hospital.

He was quite the character. One night the hospital tried to reach him by phone, but he did not answer. They asked the sheriff's deputies to go to his house and let him know it was out of order and there was an emergency case that needed attention. They knocked on his door at 3 a.m. He came to the door with a .45 automatic pistol held behind his back. Things were far less tense with the police in those days, and they thought nothing of it and had a good laugh.

Dr. Brandsma was asked by the chief of staff to audit the physicians at the Scripps Hospital in La Jolla, California. As a result, he received free medical care at Scripps. He also taught cardiology at the University of California Medical School in Irvine.

Co-author Ed and wife moved back east in 1980 after his west coast job ended. They then moved back to Carlsbad, California, in 1986, and resumed contact with Maynard and Mickie Brandsma. Ed attended Maynard's 90th birthday party in 1997.

The Brandsmas and Van Cotts spent many evenings talking about his OSS exploits, the early days of the discovery of Alzheimer's disease, his time teaching cardiac care at UC Irvine, visiting the Salk Institute, and auditing staff performance at Scripps Hospital in La Jolla, California. Maynard recommended and arranged for Mho's surgery at Scripps Clinic for a growth on Betty Van Cott's lip.

Maynard enjoyed the best cigars. His favorite was Macanudo cigars that used the finest Connecticut-grown tobacco outer wrap. They were first developed under the creative leadership of Ramon Cifuentes in 1971. Its origins started off as a Jamaican brand by the makers of Cuban Punch and branched off on its own. Today, it is produced and manufactured by General Cigar Company in the Dominican Republic. These premium cigars are available in mellow to full strengths.

Mickie and Maynard shared 34 years of marriage. He was a man of many talents in addition to his medical skill. He fished, played tennis, was a beekeeper, hunted and raised his own hunting dogs and one German shepherd who loved Ed Van Cott when he visited. After retirement, they did a lot of traveling. When Maynard became ill, Mickie lovingly cared for him at home. Mickie was the epitome of graciousness.

After Maynard died, Ed and Betty continued to visit Mickie in Mission Viejo. On one trip, gracious Mickie drove them for a visit to the Nixon Library in Yorba Linda. When Mickie died, daughter Kristin called Ed with the sad news of her death. Maynard and Mickie are buried in Big Sandy Cemetery in Choteau County, Montana. Maynard was the perfect example of a man with integrity, humility, and a wonderful friend.

We will now look at stars whom Maynard Brandsma treated from approximately 1947 to 1970.

Humphrey Bogart

Humphrey Bogart (1899-1957) became one of Maynard Brandsma's patients. Bogart was the son of a cardiopulmonary surgeon and art director. He and his friends used to put on plays near a lake in New York where he grew up. He joined the Navy in WWI and helped ferry ships back to the United States. He attended a year of college but did poorly and turned to acting.

He soon met Spencer Tracy when they co-starred in the 1930 *Up the River,* and Spencer began to call him "Bogie." John Ford directed their movie. During the production of that movie, Katharine Hepburn was having an affair with John Ford, and would later have an affair with Tracy.

In the 1930s, Bogart was unable to get much movie work and acted on the stage. He was in the Robert Sherwood play *The Petrified Forest* with British actor Leslie Howard which ran for 197 performances. When a movie was to be made of it, Howard insisted Bogart play the gangster. The studio wanted Edward G. Robinson, but Howard had choosing rights for co-stars with his contract. Bogart was so grateful that he named his only daughter Leslie Howard Bogart. His son was named Stephen because he played the role of Steve in *To Have and Have Not* where he met Lauren Bacall. He was a sentimental and grateful man.

Bogart married Helen Menken (1926-27), Mary Phillips (1928-37), Mayo Methot (1938-1945) and then married Lauren Bacall three months after his divorce. They would have his only two children. He was fond of children, a winning trait. His third wife was so jealous of his female co-stars that he avoided interaction with them by retreating to his room when there were cuts in filming. Noah Isenberg described this in his book *We'll Always Have Casablanca*.

During the filming of *Casablanca*, he was unsocial and sought no man's company. Ingrid Bergman said, "He used to stay very much to himself... I've kissed him but I don't know him!"

When he met Lauren Bacall on the set of *To Have and Have Not*, it was love at first sight. It took entire possession of him. There was something faintly fabulous in her appearance. He thought it was the beginning of a beautiful friendship, as he said in *Casablanca*. In the 1945 *The Big Sleep*, their relationship was summarized when he said, "What's wrong with you?" and she answered, "Nothing you can't fix."

Humphrey's career was so important that the American Film Institute in 1999 selected Bogart at the greatest male star of the classic American cinema. Perhaps his best roles were in 1941 *High Sierra*, 1941 *The Maltese Falcon*, 1942 *Casablanca*, 1944 *To Have and Have Not*, 1945 *The Big Sleep*, 1947 *Dark Passage*, 1948 *The Treasure of Sierra Madre*, 1948 *Key Largo*, 1950 *In a Lonely Place*, 1954 *The Caine Mutiny*, 1951 *The African Queen* (for which he earned an Oscar for Best Actor), 1954 *The Barefoot Contessa*, and 1954 *Sabrina*.

Here are quotations from 1951 *The African Queen*:

Bogart: A man takes a drop too much once in a while. It's only human nature.
Hepburn: Nature, Mr. Allnut, is what we are put in this world to rise above.
Bogart: Nobody in Africa but yours truly can get a good head of steam on that old African Queen. Fine specimen of a man, ain't I?

He and most of the cast of *Casablanca* did not know that on December 31, 1942, there was a New Year's Eve party at the White House for family and old friends. At midnight as always, President Franklin Roosevelt raised a glass of champagne and proposed a toast to the United States of America and to the formation of the United Nations two months earlier. During the evening, a movie was shown and there were few of those present who had any idea of the significance of its selection. It was Humphrey Bogart and Ingrid Bergman in *Casablanca*.

Two weeks later, the Casablanca Conference was a meeting between U.S. President Franklin D. Roosevelt and British Prime Minister Winston Churchill in the city of Casablanca, Morocco, which took place from January 14–24, 1943. They were also joined by Henri Giraud and Charles de Gaulle, who headed up opposing factions of the French resistance. Soviet Premier Joseph Stalin received an invitation but was unable to attend because the Red Army was engaged in a major offensive against the German Army at the time.

The most notable developments at the Conference were the finalization of Allied strategic plans against the Axis powers in 1943, and the policy of "unconditional surrender." It will be recalled that a phrase in the movie *Casablanca* referred to the letters of transit (hidden in the piano) as having been signed by Charles de Gaulle.[1] The timing of that conference had much to do with the early acclaim of the movie, but Bogart would die before knowing that *Casablanca* became the most famous movie of the Hollywood era, according to the American Film Institute. "We'll always have Paris," as Rick told Ilsa. And we'll always have *Casablanca*.

Humphrey loved the cinema with his whole soul. He did *The African Queen* on the radio with Greer Garson, and she handed him his Oscar for *The African Queen* in 1952. They ran into each other one day in 1956, and decided to lunch at Romanoff's restaurant in Hollywood, California. Michael Romanoff (born Hershel Geguzin in Lithuania 1890-1971) was the owner of the now defunct Beverly Hills restaurant on Rodeo Drive in the 1940s and 1950s.

Garson did not like the sound of Humphrey's terrible cough as he drank some orange juice. She insisted that Bogart go see her physician, Dr. Maynard Brandsma, an internist at the Beverly Hills Clinic. Surprisingly, he went along with her to the physician's office. Perhaps he was deeply concerned about his health. See *A Rose for Mrs. Miniver: The Life of Greer Garson* by Michael Troyan about her treatment by Dr. Maynard Brandsma.

Brandsma examined Bogart and found an inflamed esophagus. After further tests, cancer was discovered. He referred Bogart to surgeon Bert Meyer, M.D. When Dr. Brandsma told Bogart of the cancer, Humphrey said he would shoot his next picture with Bacall and then would have surgery. Maynard realized Bogart needed to know the truth, so he told him that he would die if he made the movie. He urged him to have the surgery immediately.

The actor told wife Lauren Bacall of this situation and accepted the surgery. They bore his body to surgery and a 9 ½ hour procedure was expected to totally remove all the cancer. Unfortunately, the cancer could not be completely removed. In fact, Dr. Meyer said that the cancer was so small he was sure he could get it. But after that failure, he said he would never operate on another such cancer of the esophagus if he could not do that one. Meyer also did surgery on John Wayne for his stomach cancer and tried to save Robert Kennedy's life after he was shot.

That event happened on June 5, 1968, after Senator Kennedy had given a talk. As he was taken through the hotel kitchen, Sirhan Sirhan shot him. He was first taken to one hospital then to the more adequate Hospital of the Good Samaritan. Unsure of where all the shots were in Kennedy's body, they called Dr. Bert Meyers. However, it was too late to save the Senator.

In *By Myself*, Bacall described the painful details of Bogart's decline and death. His weight loss, inability to eat solid food, the odor of decay in their bedroom and on his lips was the sad ending to his life. Brandsma talked with her many times and finally told her that they had tried everything, but the cancer was going to kill her husband. At Bacall's request, the doctor also talked with 8-year-old Stephen, who understood from that conversation that his father was going to go away. In Stephen Bogart's book about his father, *Bogart: In Search of My Father*, he also described his interactions with Dr. Brandsma.

Maynard Brandsma said: "When a man is sick, you get to know him. You find out whether he is made of soft or hard wood. I began to get fonder of Bogie with each visit. He was made of very hard wood, indeed."

Toward the end, the unhappy patient awoke from his dolor, shattered, unhinged, and powerless in the demon's grip. He knew his end was near. Two of Humphrey's last visitors were Spencer Tracy and Katherine Hepburn. They often talked of old times, but their last visit ended with Tracy and Bogart both saying "Goodbye," and knowing it was for the last time.

The end was about to come on Sunday morning. Lauren was to go to church with the children. She came back home and was talking with Humphrey until she had to go pick them up. As she left, he could have said as he did in *Casablanca,* "Kiss me. Kiss me as if it were the last time." But what he said was "Goodbye, kid. Hurry back." When she returned home, he was in a coma and the next day he died. Dr. Brandsma came that evening, confirmed he was in a coma, and warned that he might never recover. The doctor spent a very difficult time trying to help young Steve understand that his father might be gone. Lauren described their conversation in *By Myself.*

At the funeral which Brandsma attended, Lauren displayed a model of his beloved boat, the Santana, which he had bought from actor Dick Powell. Spencer Tracy was too emotional to deliver the eulogy, so Bogart's dear friend John Huston did so. Lauren Bacall had a gold whistle made to be buried with him. It was the line that brought her to attention in their first movie *To Have and Have Not* and made him pay attention. "If you want anything, just whistle."

Later, Bacall met and married actor Jason Robards, Jr. They had a child, whom she raised after their divorce, along with Stephen and Leslie Bogart. Bacall acted on stage in *Cactus Flower,* which was made into a movie with Ingrid Bergman who won a Golden Globe award for the role Bacall had played.

The boat used in *Key Largo* with Bogart and Bacall was amusingly named the *Santana.* The actual yacht named Santana (which means "holy" in Spanish) had many famous owners[2], some of whom may be of interest to movie fans, so let's round up the usual suspects:

Owner: (1939-1941) Charles Isaacs (Wife was Hungarian actress Eva Gabor)

Owner: (1941-1944) George Brent, actor
Owner: (1944-1944 3 months) Ray Milland, actor
Owner: (1944-1945) Dick & June Allyson Powell, actors
Owner: (1945-1957) Humphrey Bogart & Lauren Bacall, actors
Actors Ingrid Bergman, Richard Burton, and David Niven were frequent guests aboard Bogart's *Santana,* which he used most weekends and holidays for 10 years up to his death at age 57, and much of the sailing was around Catalina, off the California coast. Bogart raced, too, finishing first in his class in the San Clemente Island Race in 1950.
Owner: (1957-1960) Willis Short
Owner: (1960-1966) Wally Nickell, president of the Western Highway Oil
Owner: (1966-1969) William Solari, San Francisco attorney
Owner: Charlie Peet
Owner: M. Lloyd Carter, deputy attorney general of California
Owner: Ted & Tom Eden
Owner: Paul & Chrissy Kaplan (restoration after being sunk under past owner)
Owner: Wendy Schmidt, philanthropist, wife of Eric Schmidt, Executive Chairman Alphabet Inc.
Owner: Ronald Reagan & Jane Wyman, actors
Owner: Edgar Bergen ventriloquist and actor
Owner: Richard Burton, actor
Owner: David Niven, actor

Maynard Brandsma sailed on this yacht with Bogart, but Bogie could barely manage it as his illness progressed. Since

Lauren was seasick, she left the boat to Bogie who made it his male refuge center. That was the stuff his dreams were made of. He joked that the trouble with having women aboard a boat was that men couldn't pee over the side.

Notes

1. *Roosevelt and Hopkins: An Intimate History* by Robert E. Sherwood, Harper & Brothers, New York, 1948, p. 665
2. Classicyachtinfo.com

Ward Bond

Wardell Bond (April 9, 1993-November 5, 1960) was a film character actor who appeared in over two hundred movies and starred in the TV series *Wagon Train* from 1957 to 1960. He played Bert, the police officer, in 1946 *It's a Wonderful Life* and Captain Clayton in 1956 *The Searchers*.

Bond was born in Nebraska and attended the Colorado School of Mines and then the University of Southern California where he played football. He graduated from the University of Southern California (USC) in 1931 with a B.S. degree in engineering.

He and Marion Robert Morrison (John Wayne) played tackle for USC in 1926, before an injury ended Morrison's career. Bond and Wayne became life-long friends and colleagues. They and the entire USC team were hired to appear in the 1929 film *Salute,* directed by John Ford. *Salute* stars included George O'Brien, Stepin Fetchit, Frank Albertson, Ward Bond, and John Wayne was in an uncredited role as one of three midshipmen who performed a mild hazing.

John Ford appeared to be a very tough fellow but cared a lot about his friends and actors. In 1945, Bond was unable to walk due to an injury, but needed money. His wise physician Dr. Brandsma treated Ward's wounds to heal and lent him crutches and a wheelchair so he could continue work.

Ford shot the movie *They Were Expendable* with Bond in positions without walking. However, one scene required a walk so director John Ford changed the story for that character to be shot in the leg, thus he was able to use his crutches.

Ward Bond, John Wayne, and John Ford had great camaraderie with each other. They drank, ate, joshed, and talked with each other during the filming of many movies. All these men had unhealthy habits such as drinking smoking and high-fat diets. They did not care about their bodies and heart risks were not as clear as they are now with additional research. Here is a quotation from Bond and Wayne in their 1953 movie *Hondo*.

Wayne: Are you ready, Buffalo?

Bond: I was born ready.

Ward first married Hollywood socialite, Doris Sellers Child, in 1936. Was she the delicate or simply the pampered darling of doting parents? They divorced in 1944. It is drole the way we arrange marriages. No order. No method. Everything is left to chance. Ward then married his secretary and business manager, Mary Louise Meyers in 1954.

She was with him as they traveled to Dallas to see a football game between Southern Methodist University (SMU) and the University of Texas. Dr. Brandsma had warned Ward not to make the trip because of his bad heart condition. But Bond had his heart set on it. As Bond said to John Wayne in *The Searchers*, "I say we do it my way. That's an order! Yessir, but if you're wrong, don't ever give me another."

So, Bond disobeyed Brandsma's order to avoid the stress of a trip. They were in a hotel room when Bond had a massive heart attack while in the bathroom and fell against the door so that his wife could not open it. She called for help, but he died there on November 5, 1960.

In his will, Ward left everything to his wife but owned two pieces of land that he specified first option would go to John Wayne, who gave the eulogy at his funeral. Dr. Maynard Brandsma attended the service as one of the pall bearers.

John Ford

John Ford (1894-1973) was born Sean Aloysius Feeny but changed his name as did his older brother Francis Ford. He was born to an Irish immigrant family in Maine, where his father owned saloons. His Irish heritage inspired some of his movie choices. He played football in high school and followed his brother into the movies by moving to California. John was brother Francis' primary assistant and often operated the camera. He would sometimes play a bit part and was an uncredited Klansman in D. W. Griffith's 1915 *Birth of a Nation*.

He married in 1920, and had a daughter, Barbara, who was his assistant editor on five films. She married actor Robert Walker. The Fords disliked Walker, and Barbara married in private. The marriage lasted only four months. After Walker, she married actor Ken Curtis; and their son, Patrick, did movie and TV productions. Ken was a radio singer, then a cowboy singer, then an actor who appeared in movies and on the TV serial *Gunsmoke*.

John Ford liked Ken so much that he cast him in movies such as *The Quiet Man, The Searchers, Mister Roberts*, and *Rio Grande* where his rendition of "I'll Take You Home Again Kathleen" received excellent critiques. Ken became a significant help to John Ford for years by trimming the old man's toenails and doing favors. Ford might say to Curtis, "You know how I long for some music," and Ken would pour out lovely ballads. During Ford's final illness, Curtis often helped by taking directions from Dr. Maynard Brandsma and getting things Ford needed for his health.

John Ford had a five-year affair with Katharine Hepburn from 1930-1936 or so. She then had an affair of 18 months with Howard Hughes but went on to be with actor Spencer Tracy. No one ever led her to the altar. However, she visited Ford when he was dying, and he supposedly told her that he had always loved her.[1]

By the time John Ford began directing movies, his older brother's career was declining. He had worked on some 60 silent films, few of which survived. He did not begin to do westerns until *Stagecoach* in 1939, thanks to casting by brother John.

John Ford had some interesting ideas about movies. He said, "When in doubt, make a Western. It is easier to get an actor to be a cowboy than to get a cowboy to be an actor. You can speak well if your tongue can deliver the message of your heart. The main thing about directing is to photograph the people's eyes."

Stagecoach earned him seven Academy Award nominations including Best Picture and Best Director. Thomas Mitchell won Best Supporting Actor for the movie. *Stagecoach* launched John Wayne's career out of early grade B cowboy movies. Ford decided not to show up at the Academy Award ceremonies to collect any of his first three Oscars because he was fishing, or there was a war on, or he was drunk.

Ford was shot in the arm while filming WWII documentary films for the military, where he served as Rear Admiral in the U.S. Naval Reserve until 1957. Brandsma helped him tend to his arm, helped him obtain an eye patch as his vision failed, and treated his colon cancer.

Some of Ford's best movies were 1929 *Salute,* 1930 *Up the River,* 1931 *Arrowsmith,* 1935 *The Informer,* 1937 *Wee Willie Winkie,* 1939 *Young Mr. Lincoln,* 1939 *Drums Along the Mohawk,* 1940 *The Grapes of Wrath,*

1941 *Tobacco Road,* 1941 *How Green Was My Valley,* 1942 *The Battle of Midway,* 1945 *They Were Expendable,* 1946 *My Darling Clementine,* 1948 *3 Godfathers,* 1949 *She Wore a Yellow Ribbon,* 1952 *The Quiet Man,* 1953 *Mogambo,* 1955 *Mister Roberts,* 1956 *The Searchers,* 1957 *The Wings of Eagles,* 1958 *The Last Hurrah,* 1962 *The Man Who Shot Liberty Valance,* 1962 *How the West Was Won,* 1963 *Donovan's Reef,* and 1964 *Cheyenne Autumn.*

The Searchers was acclaimed by the American Film Institute in 2008 as the Greatest Western of All Time. John Ford was unique. When one is unique, one knows it. It made him kind of bossy.

John Ford had many health problems brought by an unhealthy lifestyle and wore a patch on his left eye during his last years. He had major digestive problems and often could not properly close his clothing. Maynard Brandsma, M.D. had to give him the sad news that he had colon cancer, but he continued working as long as he could. He took the news well and sat around with his old buddies, drinking, and talking about the good old days.

Ford said of doctors, "Physicians are the cobblers, rather the botchers of men's bodies; as the one patches our tattered clothes, so the other solders our diseased flesh."

He was a realist who was involved with photographing WWII. He filmed the 1942 *Battle of Midway* documentary with color footage for the U.S. Navy, because it was the turning point in the battle of the Pacific. The 18-minute film was narrated by Henry Fonda and had the voices of Jane Darwell, James Roosevelt, and Donald Crisp. Dr. Brandsma was shown the film later and thought it captured the actions extremely well having been involved in many military ships, planes, and sorties. The footage and Henry

Fonda and many well-known actors were in the 1976 movie *Midway*.

Dr. Brandsma had moved away in 1970 and was not involved in Ford's last three years of colon cancer treatment.

Notes

1. "Kate Hepburn Never Cried" Barbara Leaming, March 1, 1995. *Vanity Fair*
2. https://spartacus-educational.com/JFKhughesH.htm and bill37mccurdy.com/2010/08/13/hughes-new-howards-first-marriage/
3. https://www.nytimes.com/1077/06/26/archives/hughes-death-laid-to-massive-drug-use-illegally-obtained-medicines.html

Rock Hudson

Rock Hudson (born Roy Harold Scherer Jr. 1925-1985) was the son of an auto mechanic and telephone operator. His parents divorced when he was four and his mother married a Marine Corps officer who adopted Roy. He worked as an usher in a movie theater and developed an interest in acting, but he could not remember his lines in school plays.

After graduation from high school, he enlisted in the Navy in 1943-46. He started working odd jobs as a truck driver, and applied to the University of Southern California (USC) but was rejected due to poor grades. A talent scout found him and changed his name to Rock Hudson. He began acting in 1948 *Fighter Squadron*. He had only one line, but it took 38 takes for him to say it right.

He was hired and received coaching in acting, singing, dancing, fencing, and horseback riding. He had small parts and gradually bigger parts came along, but he always had trouble remembering dialogue. The movies cast him as a leading man in adventure films, but he played a romantic lead in 1954 *Magnificent Obsession* with Jane Wyman. It was so successful that he was then classified as a romantic star and was cast in romantic comedies with Doris Day and other stars. Here is a quotation from *Magnificent Obsession* with Jane Wyman.

> Hudson: Don't get excited. Not today.
> Wyman: May I... May I get excited tomorrow?
> Hudson: Yes.
> Wyman: And you'll be with me?
> Hudson, Yes, darling. I'll be with you tomorrow.

Wherever there is human nature, there is drama. There were rumors. There is nothing so intangible, so difficult to pin down, as the source of a rumor. Despite being gay, he made movies as a heartthrob and solidified acceptance when he married Phyllis Gates. After three years, they divorced, and she received alimony for ten years.

Maynard Brandsma, M.D. had helped him cover his homosexuality and illness by calling it allergies, liver cancer, and other things. After Brandsma's departure in 1970, other physicians were asked to do the same sort of coverup.

Hudson also made a number of TV movies and series, with the most successful being *MacMillan & Wife* opposite Susan Saint James which ran from 1971 to 1977.

One day in June 1984, a physician had to give him the unwelcome news. To avoid any kind of publicity, the physician called HIV specialist Michael Gottlieb to come over to his medical office and evaluate the celebrity. Hudson was dying of AIDS. He joined old friend Doris Day for a press conference in July 1985, which shocked viewers because he looked so gaunt and tired. At first, he was silent, standing there with his beardless face, graying hair, and his great feet.

The actor did an autobiography called *Rock Hudson: His Story* in 1986. He finally allowed the world to know that he had AIDS. That admission encouraged people to talk about the disease, accept it, and donate money to help millions of people in the future. It has been said that Rock Hudson's death gave AIDS a face. He sent this note to a September 1985 AIDS benefit:

I am not happy that I am sick. I am not happy that I have AIDS. But if that is helping others, I can at least know that my own misfortune has had some positive worth.

With his life on the wane, Rock revealed his illness. Some thought female costars who kissed him might become sick. However, Elizabeth Taylor, who had known many gay actors, purchased a bronze plaque for Hudson on the West Hollywood Memorial Walk. His former lover, Marc Christian, sued Rock's estate but because Hudson did not tell him he was sick and could have given a partner the disease. But Marc didn't get AIDS and did not win the suit.

How had he kept up this act going for so long? The audience helped because they look for and hear what they listen for. They wanted the handsome man to be a man who loved women, not men. As a youth, he struggled with shame. He was often unwilling to take advantage of his passionate reaction to certain men. He had trouble accepting himself as gay. There was something not good in his love, something ulterior about it. But now he no longer had to wear a mechanical smile with female stars in movies.

Maynard Brandsma helped him accept himself. Rock felt like a liar and a sinner and was quite certain that heaven was not for such as he. He felt sure he would go to the bad place when he died. Brandsma helped him know that God sees the heart and gladly makes allowances.

Rock yearned to be released from the lies. He had been a great actor but had covered up his secret life. Everybody wants to be somebody, to have significance, and now his admission made him an especially important person.

When he was transferred to the care of his HIV physician, Dr. Michael Gottlieb called him "the single most influential patient ever."

Carole Landis

Carole Landis (born Frances Lillian Mary Ridste 1919-1948) was an actress raised by her mother. She dropped out of high school to become a dancer. She wanted to be somebody so she renamed herself Carole Landis using the name of her favorite actress, Carole Lombard. She moved to Hollywood and began to star in movies, largely because of affairs with directors like Darryl F. Zanuck.

She first married Irving Wheeler 1934-1939, then married yachtsman Willis Hunt Jr., for less than a year. She was lovely and provocative but did not seem invested in her personal relationships. She starred in early movies such as 1937 *Broadway Melody of 1938*, 1938 *Men are Such Fools,* and 1940 *One Million B.C.* She was known as the "Ping girl" because of her curvy figure.

Because she had been in a few movies, she began to tour with other stars in the USO to perform for troops. She liked an audience and craved excitement, applause, and the adoration of lonely fellows on duty. While touring London army camps in 1942, she met and married USAF Captain Thomas Wallace.

During the war, Landis traveled more than 100,000 miles and spent more time visiting troops than any other actress. She was a popular pin-up girl with servicemen during WWII. Landis, who was nicknamed "Pride of the Yanks" by the press and "The Blonde Bomber" by soldiers, was said to teach first aid and donate blood during her spare time. She reportedly danced with 200 soldiers, invited them to her beach house on weekends, and wrote hundreds of letters to their families. Her titles included Air

Raid Warden, commander in the Aerial Nurses Corps, and honorary Colonel in the American Legion.

She pleased many men in one-night shows and relished travel, despite amoebic dysentery, malaria, and pneumonia from exotic locales in the South Pacific. Those illnesses required her to return to California for medical care. She saw Maynard Brandsma, M.D. for endometriosis and he told her that due to that condition, she would be unable to conceive. He also treated her for amoebic dysentery which she contracted during her travels with troops in Asia. His experience with such illnesses was well known.

She had visited more than 250 military bases during the war, participated in bond drives, and supported organizations like the Red Cross, the Naval Aid Auxiliary and Bundles for Bluejackets that served the armed forces. She served coffee and befriended servicemen at the Hollywood Canteen, where they could enjoy a hot meal and dance with their favorite stars free of charge.

She wrote a few magazine articles about her experiences during WWII.

They were so well received that she wrote the 1944 book *Four Jills in a Jeep*. It was made into a movie where she co-starred with Kay Francis, Martha Raye, and Mitzi Mayfair. The delightful film showed the life of such USO entertainers during the war.

Her marriage to Captain Wallace seemed to bore her, and they lived rather separate lives until their 1945 divorce. It is possible that her inability to have children disturbed both of them. She then took up with Broadway producer W. Horace Schmidlapp and they married. Again, she sought more than marriage could offer so they separated in 1947.

Her two final films were both made in the United Kingdom, 1948 *Noose* and 1948 *Brass Monkey*. This latter movie starred Herbert Lom, Ernest Thesiger, Terry-Thomas and Carole. It was about a radio personality who becomes involved in a theft and murder. Here is a quotation from the movie:

> Thesiger: The value of the three monkeys is beyond computing. They came to me as a sacred trust.
> Lom: They must be very powerful.
> Landis: I know myself too well to admit that it's over. The search will never be over until we know more about these brass monkeys.

English actor Rex Harrison was making the 1948 movie *Escape,* and they were staying in the same hotel. They began to frequent restaurants and entertainment together. Both were married but things were unsettled for them. Rex talked of divorcing his wife and that pleased Carole just as her movie career was going sour with no contracts, USO operations had ceased, and her high style of living was being cut back drastically.

When they returned to Hollywood, they still saw each other on the sly. He was then married to actress Lilli Palmer. He was called by some "Sexy Rexy." Up until the end of his life, he was a great favorite with the female sex.

Harrison seemed to have changed his mind about divorce. Carole became depressed with his mindset. She wanted to talk all this over while dining with Harrison on July 5, 1948. Her mind was in travail, she was in a state of flux. She obviously sought approval from him, but he seemed to be tossing her aside.

She was 29 with four marriages and no career opportunities seeming available. Her physical allure was gradually disappearing. Did she feel that she had nothing to look forward to? It was no consolation to know that she had set a record for the most travelled WWII actress singer.

After Harrison left her house, she took an overdose of sleeping tablets prescribed by a doctor other than Maynard Brandsma. She had already learned that Brandsma was very sparing of such prescriptions for his celebrity clients. When discovered by her maid, Rex Harrison was called over and found her suicide note.

She left this note for her mother: [1]

Dearest Mommie. I'm sorry, really sorry, to put you through this but there is no way to avoid it. I love you darling you have been the most wonderful mom ever and that applies to all our family. I love each and every one of them dearly. Everything goes to you. Look in the files and there is a will which decrees everything. Goodbye my angel. Pray for me. Your baby.

The police came to take the body. Harrison attended her funeral with his wife. Each of us is a dark mystery, a maze of conflicting passionate desires and attitudes.

Note

1. https://www.newspapers.com/clip/596137/carol_e_landis_19191948/
   For more information, see: "*Carole Landis: A Most Beautiful Girl* by Eric Gans (2008) and E. J. Fleming's *Carole Landis: A Tragic Life in Hollywood* published by McFarland in 2005.

Primula Niven (Mrs. David Niven)

British actor David Niven (1910-1983) was the son of a British Army Captain. He was sent to the Royal Military Academy at Sandhurst, graduating as second lieutenant in 1930. He joined the Highland Light Infantry and served from 1928-1933 but found it boring. In 1934, he left for Hollywood and began to star in movies. When World War II broke out in Europe, he returned to serve in the Army in 1939.

In 1940, he met Primula Rollo, daughter of Lady Kathleen Rollo and attorney William Rollo who had aristocratic backgrounds. She was working for the Women's Auxiliary Air Force (WAAF), and they married in Wiltshire, England, on September 21, 1940. He got on well with her father who served in the RAF. Her work in the WAAF was as assistant section officer in the aircraft factory near her home.

She had an unusual background because her finishing school was in Munich under Nazi Germany in December 1935. In the 1930s, many English families sent their daughters there.[1]

Following the war, David wanted to return to Hollywood to resume his career. His work there inspired Primmie to consider acting. She had a six-word role in the part in 1944 movie *English Without Tears* starring Michael Wilding, Margaret Rutherford, Lilli Palmer, and Roland Culver. It was a war-time comedy, renamed *Her Man Gilbey*.

Many of David Niven's friends met Primula and were favorably impressed. Actor Peter Ustinov said she was like a minor member of the royal family because she smiled a great deal and talked a bit like the Queen. Actor John Mills said she always let Niven be the star and claimed little attention for herself.

The Nivens had David, Jr. born in 1942 and James, born in 1945. The family planned to return to Hollywood but the enormous number of returning GIs caused a delay for Primmie and their two sons. David returned and was unfaithful according to various film stars who implied it was just his nature to be so.

Primmie and the boys arrived, and the family became active in socializing with the movie friends that Niven had made earlier. They moved next door to David's friend, Douglas Fairbanks in March 1946. Since Doug ran with the Errol Flynn crowd, the Nivens were welcomed by many other filmdom friends.

Six weeks after their arrival, they were invited to a party at the home of Tyrone Power and his French wife Arabella. They arrived and other party guests were actor Caesar Romero, former Marine pilot Arthur Little with whom Power served during the war, actress Gene Tierney with husband clothing designer Oleg Cassini, actors Richard Greene and wife Patricia Medina, and actors Rex Harrison and wife Lilli Palmer. After dinner, they decided to play a hide and seek game. Primmie Niven was "it" and the delightful young woman was to find a place to hide while the others closed their eyes and counted and then began to look for her.

Primula Niven apparently opened a door to the basement and fell down the stairs and was lying in a heap at the bottom when found. Guests carried her upstairs and laid her on a couch and she was moaning some. There was no bleeding, but she was not talking much and didn't seem to be alert. They called Dr. Maynard Brandsma whom Rex and Lilli Harrison knew. He came immediately, examined her looking intently into her eyes, and believed she should be hospitalized for observation. The ambulance arrived and took her there.

The next day, she seemed to be returning to normal and was talking some. David Niven seemed to be reassuring his friends that she would be okay. However, that second night, she stopped responding. Emergency surgery of the skull was done to visualize the traumatized brain. She stopped breathing, dying of brain lacerations. The descriptions of that dreadful evening have come from accounts by Oleg Cassini, David Niven, Gene Teirney, and Maynard Brandsma's comments to co-author Ed Van Cott.

David Niven was in shock, suddenly left with two little boys. However, some 18 months later, he met and soon married Swedish model Hjordis Genberg, and they would adopt two daughters in addition to Niven's sons.

Niven was a delightful actor and appeared in many light comedies. When he starred as Phileas Fogg in *Around the World in Eighty Days,* he said, "Crisis or not, nothing should interfere with tea!"

Perhaps David Niven's most remembered line came when he presided over the 1974 Academy Awards presentations. Suddenly, a nude man ran across the stage, with his fingers in a V-shape. The orchestra abruptly stopped. and Niven chuckled and said, "Well, ladies and gentlemen, isn't it fascinating to think that probably the only laugh that man will ever get in his life is by stripping off and showing his shortcomings?" The show continued, as it had never occurred.[2]

For more information see:

Niven, David. *Bring on the Empty Horses.* G. P. Putnam's Sons, NY, 1975.

Browne, David. "David Niven's First Wife, Primmie Niven, 1918-1946." Hjordis Genberg Niven, WordPress.com, 2019. https://hjordisniven.com/primmie-niven/

Notes

1. https://www.spiegel.de/international/europe/young-women-from-britain-in-nazi-germany-a-905617.html
2. https://collider.com/oscars-streaker-1974/

Dick Powell

Dick Powell (1904-1963) sang in church choirs and local orchestras in Little Rock, Arkansas, where he attended college for a time. He married model, Mildred Maund, from 1925-1932, and then married co-star Joan Blondell (1936-1944). He next married June Allyson in 1945 until his death.

He sang and recorded numbers for Brunswick Records in 1930 and began to star in movies in 1932. He was usually in song and dance movies until the 1940s. As he aged, he decided to be in film noir type movies and was the first actor to play Raymond Chandler's detective, Phillip Marlowe, in movies and radio. He went on to play Richard Diamond Private Detective. In those roles, he had some funny lines such as the following:

Here is a movie quotation from 1942 *Murder My Sweet* about his gun: That's just part of my clothes. I hardly ever shoot anybody with it.

A movie quotation from 1954 *Susan Slept Here:* You know, I've forgotten what seventeen-year-old emotional kids are like. I've been going out with middle-aged women; twenty, twenty-one.

June Allyson was thirteen years younger, and the old pro took her under his wing. She had a back injury in early life and transitioned from wheelchair to crutches and braces. But her cheeks glowed with the unquenchable hope of one day being able to dance. She finally did so and thanked composer Richard Rodgers for keeping her employed in musicals, according to her autobiography, *June Allyson,* published in 1982.

Dick and June often went sailing in the yacht called *Santana,* which they sold after a year to Humphrey Bogart in 1945. Powell became terribly busy directing and producing movies and made two films with June.

He directed a movie financially backed by Howard Hughes in 1956 called *The Conqueror* with John Wayne, Susan Hayward, and Agnes Moorhead. It was filmed in St. George, Utah, near a site in Nevada where 11 atomic bombs were tested the year before they began filming. It was later learned that instead of being safe as the government had told Hughes, it was contaminated by nuclear fallout.

After thirteen brutal weeks of hot sun and flash floods, they returned to California, and Hughes shipped 60 tons of the soil to their Hollywood set for final takes, causing even more radioactive exposure.

An article about that location by James Rice[1] was published recently in the *Western Historical Quarterly,*

> Harry, a 32-kiloton shot in May of 1953, was the dirtiest atmospheric detonation ever conducted at the Nevada Test Site in terms of population exposure to radioactive contamination. Fallout descended upon St. George, Utah, and residents were instructed to shelter in place for approximately two hours. Harry not only illustrated the inadequacies of the Atomic Energy Commissions management of offsite fallout, but also called into question modernist assumptions of the command and control of nature.

There were rumors about the earlier test site, so John Wayne was photographed using a Geiger counter as a joke, but it made so much noise, they thought it was broken.

After filming, the 220-person cast, and crew members started getting cancer. Powell, Hayward, Wayne, Pedro Armendariz, Lee Van Cleef, and Dick Powell died of cancer. Out of the group, some 91 persons contracted cancer causing many deaths.

Hughes could not be blamed because the government had said the site was safe. However, his constant fiddling with details on all his films prolonged the making of the movie and exposure to radiation.

Hughes wanted to make this movie, but it was poorly received and won awards as one of the worst movies ever produced. Wayne as Genghis Khan was miscast saying lines such as these: "There are moments fer wisdom, then I listen to you and there are moments fer action. Then I listen to my blood. I feel this Tartar woman is fer me, and my blood says take her!'" Susan Hayward said: "The Conqueror? Mighty armies cannot stop him. But one touch of my lips... Yes, he captured me, but he cannot tame me." Agnes Moorhead said: "My son has won the world. Still, he must conquer that red-headed Jezebel."

Howard Hughes felt guilty about the whole thing. He called the choice of the film's shooting location the worst mistake of his life. This movie spelled the end of RKO and Hughes never again produced movies. He bought up all copies of *The Conqueror* and it was not shown again for 21 years until Universal bought the rights to the film in 1979. As Hughes became sicker in his terminal illness, he obsessively watched this movie almost daily.

The movie studio that had begun with the RKO (Keith-Albee-Orpheum) theater chain and Joseph P. Kennedy merged in 1928 under the control of the Radio Corporation of America (RCA). After producing eleven movies, Kennedy wanted to get out of the movie business and stepped down in 1932. His paramour, Gloria Swanson and newcomer William Holden were in 1929 *The Trespasser* and 1930 *What a Widow,* and she was in *Queen Kelly,* directed by Erich von Stroheim.

Howard Hughes took over RKO in 1948. Hughes first act was to fire half the staff and favor certain actors like Jane Russell and Faith Domergue. Hughes caused years of disarray and decline until he sold RKO to General Tire and Rubber Company in 1955.

The House Un-American Activities Committee began hearings on Communism in the movie industry. That caused many to be fired or never again employed whether they named suspected communists or not. By 1952, Hughes was fighting off lawsuits by those he fired. Dick Powell said "RKO's contract list is down to three actors and 127 lawyers."

Powell knew his years as an actor were dwindling so he, Charles Boyer, David Niven, and Ida Lupino founded Four Star Television. He hosted the *Dick Powell Zane Grey Theater* on CBS from 1956 to 1961.

He began to have physical symptoms that he thought were allergies and went to see his internist Dr. Maynard Brandsma. He had seen Brandsma for lung damage due to years of smoking. Brandsma thought it was profoundly serious and referred him to the Medical Center at the University of California in Los Angeles. He was found to have a combination of problems with cancer tumors in his neck and chest, lung cancer, and lymphoma which is a cancer in the cells of his lymph nodes. His symptoms included fatigue, shortness of breath, swollen lymph nodes, chest pain, and feeling full after eating very little food.

Radiation treatments reduced the size of the tumors, and he was able to keep working for a while. However, the disease progressed, and he lapsed into a coma on New Year's Day of 1963 and died the next day. Wife June Allyson asked for no eulogy, but many stars turned out for the beloved actor.

June Allyson continued to act and did various charity events. She became the spokesperson for Depends, which allowed urinary incontinence to be dealt with in a caring manner. After Dick's death, she married Dick's barber and later married David Ashrow until her death.

Her lifelong interest in medical research caused her to be appointed by President Ronald Reagan to the Federal Council on Aging, and she actively supported fundraising for various medical causes and for the museums of her friends, James Stewart, and Judy Garland. For more information, see her book *June Allyson* by June Allyson.

James Rice[1] was published in the *Western Historical Quarterly*, Volume 54, Issue 3, Autumn 2023, pp. 222-238, https://doi.org/10.1093/whq/whad081.

John Wayne

John Wayne (1907-1979) was born Marion Robert Morrison. When he was five, his mother told him that his new brother had been named Robert after Grandpa Brown. Little Marion was confused. He was Marion Robert Morrison and his mother had even been calling him "Bobby." But now they were going to call his baby brother Bobby. For his mother, the new baby was going to be special, and she wanted him to have her father's name.

For almost sixty years, she would shower attention on Bobby. She did not like Marion (who became John Wayne) and he knew it. Her negative attitude haunted him. He spent many decades trying to please her, but she would not be pleased. He, therefore, had trouble trusting women and men became his soulmates. This information came from Rand Roberts and James Olson who wrote about John Wayne.[1]

His father first tried to run a Rexall pharmacy but failed and moved to farming in Iowa. Marion helped with various farm chores and rode a horse to school each day. Horseback riding in very early movies was a skill he thought he knew. But there, his double stuntman Yakima Canutt, coached and guided him into being a successful screen cowboy who made his way into our hearts.

John Wayne played college football at the University of Southern California on a full sports scholarship. Ward Bond was a college football teammate. However, John injured his collarbone on a beach accident and lost his scholarship. But the relationship between Bond and Wayne continued up to their deaths.[2]

As he moved on to success in movies, he sent his mother and her new husband on worldwide tours, but she was never happy or thankful. He tired of how she tried to control him and his father. He chose to involve himself with directors, co-stars, and others who could be true and loyal. In his love life, he chose to be with women he could control. Those women included his three wives and his secretary who was his final lover. However, he fell for some extraordinarily strong women whom he could not control such as Marlene Dietrich, Merle Oberon, and Maureen O'Hara.

After simple Westerns, he joined John Ford's crew. He was impressed because Ford had actually met Western lawman Wyatt Earp through his actor friend, Harry Carey. Earp and movie cowboy Tom Mix used to hang around with Ford to go over ideas for movies. For example, Earp told Ford exactly what happened in the gunfight at the OK Corral, and Ford depicted it in 1946 *My Darling Clementine*. Lawman Earp (1848-1929) told Ford that he never used a gun except as a last resort. John Wayne learned about Earp's code and told his crew on *The Shootist* he didn't want his character to shoot anybody in the back.[3]

After John's frustrating mother, he chose to marry Latin women believing they cared more about simple things like marriage, family, children, and home.

In 1933, 26-year-old John married Josephine Saenz, the daughter of a Panamanian Consul in Los Angeles. They had Michael in 1934, Mary in 1936, Patrick in 1939, and Melinda in 1940. John's wife was a strict Catholic. She did not believe in birth control and after they had four children and wanted no more, she would not sleep with him. Instead, she invited her mother to share her bed and they talked Spanish all the time leaving him out of things. Fortunately, he loved children and spent time with them when he could.

He married again in 1946 to Esperanza Baur, the daughter of a madame who had brothels. He saw this spitfire dancing and wanted her. However, when she learned he did not want her to have a movie career, she began drinking alcohol and using sleeping pills. She cut her wrists at one point, believing that he was involved with his female co-stars. Then one day he came home to find her drunk and holding a gun at the door to shoot him. That was the end of their marriage.

He married his third wife, Pilar Pallete, in 1954. She was a more sophisticated lady, and a good tennis player who hoped to involve him in sports. He was unhappy with marriage and busy at many sites so was home little. He was involved with several affairs and business deals in Arizona. The couple finally separated in 1973 because he had become romantically involved with his secretary Pat Stacy.

Pat nursed him through his final illnesses and wrote 1983 *Duke: A Love Story*. The book is very explicit about his suffering through illness. He did not divorce Pilar and she also wrote *John Wayne, My Life with the Duke*. The artistic woman was exceedingly kind in describing John and went on to have a restaurant and write cookbooks.[4]

One of Wayne's paramours was actress Merle Oberon (1911-1979). They enjoyed an off and on affair from 1938 to 1947. They both had very unusual backgrounds. John undoubtedly shared his carefully with her. She may have shared hers with him, but she had told others that she came from Australia.

Let us go back in time. A woman of Eurasian and Maori descent from Ceylon had a lover in Bombay, India. He was an English railway engineer. He raped a child of hers who was 11 or 12 years old. The infant born to the 12-year-old was Merle. So, her grandmother raised her daughter and granddaughter to believe they were sisters about 11 years apart. They did not learn until their mother died that they were mother and daughter but were always remarkably close. Merle's slightly Asian face attracted many people when she entered show business.

Her affair of nine years with John Wayne offered only occasional romance when the two chanced secret meetings.[5]

She married English director Alexander Korda 1939-1945 who changed her name from Merle Thompson to Merle Oberon. She next married camera man Lucien Ballard 1945-1949, industrialist Bruno Pagliai in 1957-1973, and Dutch actor Robert Wolders in 1975 until her death. He was 25 years her junior. Often a nice respectable woman of age leaves a whole family in order to link her life with a younger man, considerably her junior.

Wayne starred with Marlene Dietrich in 1940 *Seven Sinners*, 1942 *The Spoilers*, and 1942 *Pittsburgh*. John Wayne carried on a three year on-off affair with Dietrich whom he called the most "intriguing" woman he'd ever known. Wayne obsessed over how Dietrich risked death to perform for frontline troops during World War II. She crossed into enemy territory alongside General George Patton and smuggled Jews out to safety. John's affair with Merle brought his first marriage to a close.[6]

Wayne's affair with Marlene Dietrich caught the attention of the F.B.I. Director J. Edgar Hoover who wanted his people to check whether Dietrich was a Nazi sympathizer. She and John Wayne were found to be extremely opposed to Nazis. John Wayne and Hoover exchanged letters and supported each other in their work.

After the attack on Pearl Harbor by the Japanese, Wayne went to register for the military and found that he was not eligible as a married man with four children. He did USO tours in 1942 and 1943. He had recently finished his first big movie—*Stagecoach,* and his big-time career lay ahead of him.

The remarkable red-haired Dublin lass, Maureen O'Hara, hit it off with John Wayne and they starred in five movies together. By that time, Wayne was losing so much hair that he started using a hairpiece and Maureen kidded him about that. They were in 1950 *Rio Grande,* 1952 *The Quiet Man,* 1957 *The Wings of Eagles,* 1963 *McLintock,* and 1971 *Jake,* and the first three were directed by John Ford. Maureen and John were friends from their first movie to the end of his life. She and Duke had such fun together. Here are two scenes in *The Quiet Man* where O'Hara is Mary Kate Danaher and Wayne is Thornton:

> O'Hara: I have a fearful temper. You might as well know about it now instead of findin' out about it later. We Danahers are a fighting people.
> Wayne: I can think of a lot of things I'd rather do to one of the Danahers, Miss Danaher.
> O'Hara: Shhh, Mr. Thornton! What will Mr. Flynn be thinkin'?
> Wayne: If anybody had told me six months ago that today I'd be in a graveyard in Innisfree with a girl like you that I'm just about to kiss, I'd have told 'em…
> "O'Hara: Oh, but the kisses are a long way off yet!
> Wayne: Huh?
> O'Hara: Well, we just started a'courtin,' and next month we start the walkin' out, and the month after

that there'll be the threshin' Parties, and the month after that...
Wayne: Nope.
O'Hara: Well, maybe we won't have to wait that month...
Wayne: Yup.
O'Hara: ... or for the threshin' parties..
Wayne: Nope.
O'Hara: ...or for the walkin' out together...
Wayne: No.
O'Hara:... and so much the worse for you, Sean Thornton, for I feel the same way about it myself! [They kiss. Thunder rolls]

Usually, Wayne passed his time between takes on the movie set by playing chess. He was excellent and played with others such as Marlene Dietrich, Kirk Douglas, Dean Martin, Roger Ebert, and Rock Hudson. He, like Humphrey Bogart, was particularly good at chess. But when he was around the strong-minded red head, their personal charisma was extraordinary. Their chemistry was clear to see in movies as they heartily said their words to each other. Despite both of their spouses, they saw a lot of each other. Their hanky-panky was mostly reserved by time at the Arizona ranch Wayne owned.

In 1964, Dr. Maynard Brandsma had to tell John he had cancer of the left lung which had spread to his ribs. He referred Wayne to the same surgeon, Dr. Bert Meyer, who had operated on Humphrey Bogart. Meyer taught at the University of Southern California as did Brandsma and both mentored many physicians. Meyer also assisted in Senator Robert Kennedy's fight for life on June 6, 1968.

Wayne's operation removed his left lung and four ribs. It took him some time to recuperate. Brandsma told him to follow a healthy diet because he was a devil-may-care kind of guy. He did stop smoking cigarettes but substituted small cigars. He had to have oxygen on the movie set as he recovered.

He had trouble with his weight but was told by *True Grit* director Henry Hathaway not to diet because the character was a sloppy drunk. In 1970, John Wayne received his only Academy Award which was for Best Actor in *True Grit* for a character with a patch over his eye. At the Award presentation, he said: "Wow, if I'd known that, I'd have put that patch on thirty-five years earlier." When he got back to work on a movie set the next morning, all the crew had their backs turned to him. But in a minute, they turned around and all were wearing eye patches, including the horses.

During the last fifteen years of his life, beginning with lung cancer, Wayne had various health problems. After he beat lung cancer, he never followed a healthy diet. We will never know whether the experience with Dick Powell's movie *The Conquerer* where Wayne played Ghenghis Khan near atomic blast sites making the movie had anything to do with his cancer.

At the point where John was becoming very ill, dear friend Maureen O'Hara visited him when he lived with Pat Stacy. Maureen imagined she would be there only one day, but he was so enthusiastic and did so much better in her presence, she stayed a week. She washed her one set of clothing every night so that he could see her looking fresh each morning.

Another physician who took over after Dr. Brandsma left in 1970 told Wayne to get his life in order because his cancer had spread, and he could not lick this one. He made *The Shootist* in 1976 while being in pain throughout the filming.

He had starred with *Shootist* co-star Lauren Bacall in the 1955 *Blood Alley* movie. Bogart visited the set of *Blood Alley* during the filming. John Wayne hardly knew him but was the first to send flowers when he learned of Bogart's cancer that year.

The crew of old friends (James Stewart, Richard Boone, Scatman Crothers, Hugh O'Brian, and new friend Ron Howard) worked with less pay than usual because they thought *The Shootist* would be John Wayne's last film. Even old almost deaf pal James Stewart, who missed some cues for lack of hearing, wanted to be near him.

Wayne's next big medical problem was his heart. He had a heart valve that was misfunctioning and causing shortness of breath and other symptoms. In 1978, they performed a heart valve replacement. In January 1979, he had what was expected to be routine gall bladder surgery, but that found cancer cells in several places. The primary tumor was the pancreas, and they had to remove his cancerous stomach in a 9½ hour surgical procedure.

On April 9, 1979, he was invited to the Academy Awards to award the Oscar for Best Picture. When he walked on stage, the audience gasped as the saw the thin man proceeding to the microphone. They burst out in a tremendous ovation. There he stood, fixed in thought for a moment. Then he answered their ovation saying, "That's just about the only medicine a fellow could ever need."

On April 20, 1979, he was hospitalized for a bronchial condition brought on from flu. He was again hospitalized May 3, 1979, to remove an intestinal obstruction at the

UCLA Medical Center. President Jimmy Carter stopped in to visit him for about fifteen minutes on May 5, 1979. Carter said: "I want you to know that you have the love, affection, and prayers of not only everybody in our nation, but of millions of persons around the world."

There are things that cannot be hurried, like nature and old people. So, he lingered on for a very painful period of time. Lauren Bacall wrote him a letter on May 7, 1979, a month before his death. Here is what she said:

Dear Duke,

This letter has been on its way to you for months. You have been so very much in my thoughts. I have never been able to tell you how much you standing up for me in *Blood Alley* days meant to me. I wanted to say it on *The Shootist*. Never could somehow. I know how difficult that film was for you.

You have the guts of a lion. I do admire you more than I can say. It was good to see you at the Academy Awards night. I'm being inarticulate. I want you to know how terrific you are. You give more than you know.

I send you much love. Constant thoughts. Betty.

John Wayne converted to Catholicism on his death bed at his home. His first wife had introduced him to the Catholic world and dragged him to church events and fundraisers. One of their daughters, Melinda, had a son who became a priest, Father Matthew Munoz was fourteen when his grandfather died. He described that conversion which was done by an archbishop. Munoz said, "He wanted to be baptized and become Catholic. It was wonderful to see him come to the faith and to leave that witness for our whole family."[7]

Most people think of John Wayne in connection with Monument Valley which many call "John Wayne country." He made five movies there: *Stagecoach* 1939, *Fort Apache* 1948, *She Wore a Yellow Ribbon* 1949, *Rio Grande* 1950, and *The Searchers* 1956.

But John Wayne country was elsewhere in Arizona. He named it *Red River* after his favorite movie. Louis and Alice Johnson managed Wayne's cotton and cattle farms in Arizona. He would often visit when he needed to drop some weight for an upcoming movie role. This place had the power to beguile him, to relax his body, and to make him glad to be alive.

Alice followed a plan from a diet book, but the key was that they specially designed John's bathroom with mirrors on every surface except ceilings and floors. That way, he was able to see his body from every angle to drop his weight. Their relationship continued until John died.

Notes

1. Washingtonpost.com/wp-srv/style/longterm/books/chap1/wayne.htm)
2. https://outsider.com/entertainment/wagon-train-ward-bond-played-college-football-john-wayne-what-to-know-western-stars-sports-careers/
3. https://www.wideopencountry.com/wyatt-earp/
4. https://classiccountrymusic.com/meet-all-of-john-waynes-wives-including-1-who-tried-to-shoot-him-dead/

5. www.hollywoodsgoldenage.com/actors/merle-oberon.html
6. cheatsheet.com/entertainment/john-wayne-called-marlene-dietrich-intriguing-woman-ever-known.html
7. https://web.archive.org/web/20111006041651/

CHAPTER FOUR
Ralph Greenson. M.D.

Ralph Greenson (born Romeo Samuel Greenschpoon 1911-1979) was a psychiatrist and psychoanalyst born to a Russian Jewish couple. His father was a general physician and he and twin sister Juliet were named by their parents after *Romeo and Juliet*, the tragedy of warring families by William Shakespeare. He was brought up in New York, and his twin became a pianist who married lawyer Milton Rudin.

Romeo studied at Columbia University School of Medicine in New York but a quota system for Jews was in place, so he enrolled at the University of Bern in Switzerland for his medical training. He quickly learned German to study there from 1930 to 1934. In Bern, he met Hildegard Troesche, and they married in 1935 in Los Angeles.

He studied Freudian psychology in Vienna, Austria, Sigmund Freud's homeland. He underwent psychoanalysis with one of Freud's disciples, Dr. Wilhelm Stekel, beginning in 1935.

Psychoanalysts see most patients three or more times a week for approximately an hour each visit. The patient relaxes on couch as the analyst sits behind taking notes. Analysis usually takes months to years as the patient tries to achieve his goals of self-understanding. At best, it enlarges people, helps them see their potential, taps into their passions, addresses character flaws, and focuses on their strengths.

Romeo became a close friend of Freud's youngest daughter, psychoanalyst Anna Freud. He and wife Hildi returned to the U.S. in 1937, where he changed his name to Ralph Greenson. He entered the Los Angeles Psychoanalysis Institute where he met Otto Fenichel, with whom he continued his psychoanalysis.

Greenson began his national service during WWII in 1942, treating soldiers at the Veterans Hospital in New York. After a serious collision which damaged his face and arm, he was discharged from military service and was named to lead the neuropsychiatric department at the Air Force convalescent hospital at Fort Logan in Colorado. Promoted to Captain, he ran a unit designated as "operational fatigue." Those words were later changed to "post-traumatic stress disorder" or PTSD.

Greenson's work with GIs who had been close to danger was commemorated in a movie where Gregory Peck played the role of psychiatrist Greenson in the 1963 movie *Captain Newman*. The movie also starred Tony Curtis, one of Dr. Greenson's patients in real life.

When Greenson returned to civilian life, he started another psychoanalysis with Frances Deri, as he settled in to be a psychiatrist in Los Angeles. She was a psychoanalyst from Vienna who fled the Nazis with about 90 other analysts. She and Erik Erikson, who underwent psychoanalysis with Anna Freud, began a new California psychoanalytic society.

That study group was open to all interested medical and academic individuals, which included psychologists, social workers, and scientists. Robert Oppenheimer, the famous nuclear physicist, attended these meetings at the University of California.[1]

Dr. Greenson saw many famous patients who were movie stars. Greenson was unusual for a psychoanalyst because he often gave patients medicines like barbiturates or sedatives rather than relying upon talking therapy alone to help patients.

Greenson authored papers on unusual subjects such as gambling, transference in therapy, and difficulties with borderline patients who might have experienced unusual family circumstances. All who were in training to do psychoanalytic therapy paid much attention to his book *The Technique and Practice of Psychoanalysis* published in 1967. He gave talks at conferences for psychoanalysts, psychiatrists, and psychologists who listened carefully to figure out when he might be talking about patients like Marilyn Monroe. His talks were always well attended and discussed in detail at each table of attendees.

He wrote and spoke about the struggle for patients to identify with someone in 1954. He explained that we take someone into our selves called incorporation or introjection. He used that term in connection with Marilyn Monroe and other patients whom he occasionally gave medicines to, as if to take into their bodies a little bit of their therapist to calm them down or help them act like a person they respected. That was a view of medicine not shared by all psychoanalysts.[2]

Ralph Greenson frequently corresponded with Anna Freud about those psychoanalysts who were deviating away from Freudian techniques. He may have described those deviants unfairly according to Douglas Kirsner who published an essay about this in December 2005 in the *Psychoanalytic Review*, 92 (6). It was entitled "Politics

Masquerading as Science: Ralph Greenson, Anna Freud, and the Klein Wars." His point was that the politics of Anna and Ralph in discussing their critics were not scientific but personal.

Kirsner was not the only one who felt that practices by Anna and Sigmund Freud were not always correct. Alan A. Stone, M.D. wrote "How Freud Worked: First-Hand Accounts of Patients" published June 1, 1998.[3] Stone pointed out that Freud violated some of his own technical rules by analyzing some patients for free, socializing with patients he liked, analyzing several members of the same family, and trying to recruit some patients to become psychoanalysts.

Such practices gave Anna and Ralph Greenson room to violate rules themselves. It was the philosophy, "Do as I say and not as I do." Other analysts rallied around Anna and Greenson and pointed out that the analyst must be a human being who cares about patients.

Since psychoanalysis is not supposed to involve patients outside of normal office hours, it was surprising that he had some patients come to his house for meals, such as Monroe. He explained that analysts had to step beyond talking therapy for some patients who did not have a normal childhood. He tried to explain his actions by saying that some patients needed to see a loving family and demonstrated that by involving his wife and children.

That practice violated rules of therapy seemingly established by Sigmund Freud and later analysts. But Sigmund had violated those rules when he did analysis with his own daughter, Anna. She in turn, violated those rules by asking some patients, like Marilyn Monroe, to donate major funding for museums and therapy institutions that she had some role in controlling. Greenson was not the only physician who was violating ethical rules with patients, as we will see with some others doctor described later.

It was daunting to trainees to learn that Ralph Greenson and Anna Freud cajoled some patients into donations that were far outside the realm of objective counseling. Marilyn Monroe was one of many early patients who were used in unfortunate ways by her analysts. Integrity is essential for those who would influence others. It shows basic goodness, moral character, and honesty.

Monroe needed someone with integrity to help her curb her impulses to act without considering the results. Her numerous sexual improprieties had cost her a sense of self-respect. Toward the end of her life, she tried to regain self-respect by becoming Mrs. John Kennedy. That hope disappeared just before her suicide.

Ralph Greenson had cardiac problems and was given a pacemaker in 1970. He suffered a stroke and was unable to talk for several weeks in 1974. He died in 1979, having held his silence about Marilyn Monroe for years after her death. See more on Ralph Greenson papers.[4]

Notes

1. https://www.encyclopedia.com/psychology/dictionaries-thesauruses-pictures-and-press-releases/san-francisco-psychoanalytic-society-and-institute/) "Inside the Center: The Life of J. Robert Oppenheimer by Ray Monk review and https://www.theguardian.com/books/2012/nov/16/ihnside-cedntre-robert-oppenheimer-ray-monk-review) Also, see the movie *Oppenheimer* for Oppie's remarks about psychoanalysis and psychology.
2. https://journals.sagepub.com/doi/10.1177/000306515400200202)
3. https://ajp.psychiatryonline.org/doi/10.1176/ajp.155.6.851)
4. https://www.library.ucla.edu/special-collections

Tony Curtis

Tony Curtis was born Bernard Schwartz (1925-2010) in New York City. His family were Hungarian Jews, and his father was a tailor. His mother and brother were hospitalized for schizophrenia. When he was eight, he and brother Julius were placed in a state orphanage because their parents couldn't feed them. The boys were often attacked by antisemites at that site. Julius died when he was hit by a truck. Curtis joined a neighborhood gang who were truant from school and stole items from the local variety store.[1]

A friendly neighbor helped the handsome lad by sending him to a Boy Scout camp where he learned to work and continued school. The figure of this half-grown teen was a masterpiece of nature. It not only pleased the eye but evoked the neighbor's sympathy.

He was in a school stage play at age 16. Admiration for his performance caused him to consider movies. He went to see movies and used male stars as role models for how to do something significant. He enlisted in the U.S. Navy to be in a submarine, having been inspired by actor Cary Grant in the 1943 *Destination Tokyo* and Tyrone Power in the 1943 *Crash Drive* movies. He served aboard the *USS Proteus*, until the end of WWII. He was a signalman 3rd Class from 1943-1945 and was awarded campaign medals and a WWII Victory Medal.

He then attended City College of New York on the GI bill and studied acting at the New School in Greenwich Village along with Walter Matthau, Bea Arthur, Harry Belafonte, and Rod Steiger. He was discovered by Joyce Selznick, a notable talent scout and niece of movie producer David O. Selznick.

He dated girls including Marilyn Monroe briefly, and began work at Universal Pictures, changing his name to Anthony Curtis. He didn't expect to become a big star, but he didn't want to return home as a failure. He wanted to be somebody. He was uncredited in several movies but finally was named Tony Curtis in some Westerns such as 1950 *Sierra,* 1950 *Winchester '73,* and 1951 *Kansas Raiders.* As he began to receive fan letters, he was given a starring role in 1951 *The Prince Who Was a Thief* and 1952 *Flesh and Fury.*

He married Janet Leigh (1951-1962) and they starred in 1953 *Houdini* and 1954 *Shield of Falworth.* Both became major stars. He joined Burt Lancaster in 1956 *Trapeze.* The couple then formed their own film production company called Curtleigh Productions in 1955. They had children Kelly and Jamie Lee Curtis. Burt Lancaster had enjoyed working with Tony and asked him to play in 1957 *Sweet Smell of Success.* Curtis received excellent reviews which began to convince him that he wasn't just another pretty face.

Tony expected to enjoy starring in 1959 *Some Like It Hot* with Marilyn Monroe, Jack Lemmon, George Raft and Joe E. Brown. He and many others were miserable as Monroe was late, forgot lines, was difficult to work with, and delayed production with her many eccentricities.

He gladly starred in 1959 *Operation Petticoat* with idol Cary Grant.

The Curtis marriage was troubling, so Janet and Tony separated. He took up with young co-star Christine Kaufmann in 1962 *Taras Bulba.* He married the Austrian German, some 20 years younger, until 1968 and they had two daughters.

In 1963, he starred in *Captain Newman, M.D.,* with Gregory Peck who played the role of Ralph Greenson,

M.D. The movie about the psychoanalyst was made by Ralph's friend, Leo Rosten. During WWII, Greenson ran the neuropsychiatric hospital and the movie crew also included Robert Duval, Angie Dickinson, Eddie Albert, and Bobby Darin. The movie displayed GIs who had post-traumatic stress disorders due to their close calls on the military frontlines. Here is a quotation from the movie:

> Peck: You mustn't confuse sadness with depression.
> Curtis: Is there any difference? Can a man look sad and still be happy?
> Peck: Yes.
> Curtis: Example?
> Peck: You.

The therapy offered by Dr. Ralph Greenson to Tony Curtis has never been discussed by either party. It is likely that they discussed his difficult early life and fear of schizophrenia, his relationships, heartbreaks, and struggle with the loss of his attractiveness. He may have discussed his use of drugs and alcohol which threatened his career. He was found to have marijuana on a flight to London and was arrested. He would lose a 23-year-old son to a heroin overdose in 1994.[2]

Curtis' marriage and his career waned, and he divorced Kaufmann and married Leslie Allen from 1968 to 1982, with whom he had two sons. Later, he married another young lady, Andrea Savio from 1984 to 1992, then married Lisa Deutsch from 1993 to 1994, and finally married Jill Vanderberg, 45 years younger in 1998 until his death in 2010. Perhaps his disgust over his own aging body was mollified by a pretty young woman who loved and complimented him.

He starred in many movies but turned to television in the 1970s. He had enjoyed painting throughout his life and became more active in painting in the 1980s. Curtis had problems with alcohol and drug abuse with cocaine and went to the Betty Ford Clinic for treatment in the mid-1980s with good success.

He and daughter Jamie Lee Curtis studied their Hungarian Jewish heritage and helped refinance the building of the Great Synagogue in Budapest, Hungary, the largest synagogue in Europe. It was built in 1859 but suffered damage during WWII, and that was repaired through their efforts. In 1998, he also founded the Emanuel Foundation for Hungarian Culture which aimed to restore and preserve synagogues and the 1300 Jewish cemeteries in Hungary, dedicated to the 600,000 Jewish victims of the Holocaust in Hungary.[3]

When he died of lung problems from smoking and asthma, actor Kirk Douglas and singer Phyllis McGuire were honorary pallbearers.

Notes

1. https://web.archive.org/web/20110907041843/ and http: www.biography.com/articles/Tony- Curtis-9263844
2. https://www.upi.com/Archives/1994/07/05/Actor-Tony-Curtis-son-dies-on-Cape-Cod/3868773380800/ UPI. July 5, 1994.)
3. https://web.archive.org/web/20121104205238/http:www. highbeam.com/doc/1P2-3892380.html Chicago Sun-Times. June 29, 1988.

Celeste Holm

Celeste Holm (1917-2012) was the only child of a Norwegian businessman and portrait artist mother. She traveled and attended schools in the Netherlands, France, and the U.S. She studied drama at the University of Chicago before becoming an actress in the 1930s.

She appeared on stage with greats such as Leslie Howard, Gene Kelly, and was in the musical *Oklahoma* in 1943. She signed a movie contract in 1946 and acted in movies such as *Gentlemen's Agreement* with Gregory Peck, *All About Eve* with Marilyn Monroe and Bette Davis, and *High Society* with Frank Sinatra. She was active on television as well. She received awards and was a spokesperson for UNICEF during the 1990s. She was inducted into the Scandinavian American Hall of Fame in 1995.

After 1947 *Gentlemen's Agreement*, she asked for a salary raise and Darryl Zanuck fired her saying she was difficult to work with. She was immediately hired by director Joe Mankiewicz, who paid her three times her contract salary. She won Best Supporting Actress for her role in that film.

While making 1950 *All About Eve,* a feud developed between Bette Davis and Celeste Holm. The first morning of shooting, a chipper Holm walked onto the set with Bette and said, "Good morning. Isn't it a beautiful day." Bette said, "Oh shit, good manners." Holm did not speak to her except for their movie dialogue after that. She must have thought "Why did she spoil it and turn the morning greeting into the ugly and commonplace piece of life?" These slights and criticisms by others may have been part of the conversations with Ralph Greenson.

Celeste first married movie and TV actor/director Ralph Nelson from 1936 to 1939. She next married English auditor Francis Davis from 1940 to 1945. Her third marriage was to a public relations director for an airline, A. Schuyler Dunning, from 1946 to 1953. She then married actor Wesley Addy from 1961 until his death in 1996. Her last marriage was to a man 46 years younger, opera singer Frank Basile.

She worked with Ralph Greenson for a short period and after treatment became a friend. One day when he invited her to dinner, she was shocked to find that Marilyn Monroe was there but was currently in treatment with Dr. Greenson. After dinner, Celeste went walking with Greenson. She took him to task saying he never asked her to come for dinner during treatment. He responded, "You weren't that sick... This child has no frame of reference. She has no idea what the goal is."

Greenson tried to explain to many, including Anna Freud, that he was showing Monroe what life was like in a family, which she had never seen. He was playing at being Marilyn's family and his wife and children were playing like this was family life.[1]

Holm was deeply involved in many organizations that helped people such as Jews, the retarded, medical and mental illnesses, and others where she used her stardom to bring attention to the needs of people. She was in the 2002 edition of the Marquis *Who's Who of American Women*.

In 1950 *All About Eve,* after actor Hugh Marlowe questioned her cynicism, she said:

Holm: That cynicism you refer to, I acquired the day I discovered I was different from little boys!

In 1948 *The Gentlemen's Agreement* about the lack of acceptance of Jews by Caucasians, there was a conversation about Jews between Curt Conway and Celeste Holm:

Conway: "What? Now, Green, don't get me wrong. Why, some of my best friends are Jews."

Holm: "And some of your other best friends are Methodists, but you never bother to say that."

Celeste began to have memory loss and she was in poor health for some time before she died. She was survived by her sons, and her fifth husband.[3]

Notes

1. http://moresketchynotes.blogspot.com/2009/08/century-of-self-part-2-engineering-of.html
2. https://www.closerweekly.com/posts/all-about-eve-secrets-bette-davis-and-celeste-holms-feud-plus-more/
3. blog.everlasting-star.net/tag/Gregory-ratoff/

Vivien Leigh

Vivien Leigh, born Vivian Mary Hartley 1913-1967, in Darjeeling, British India, was the only child of a British broker and his wife. Her father gave her the works of Hans Christian Andersen, Lewis Carroll, Rudyard Kipling, and mythology to read during her childhood.

A friend in London where she was sent to a convent was future actress Maureen O'Sullivan. Vivien attended schools in Europe and when her father learned of her interest in acting, he sent her to the Royal Academy of Dramatic Art in London.

There she met Herbert Leigh Holman, a barrister 13 years older, who wanted her to marry him and end her tawdry theater life. They had a daughter whom she never cared much about, but then she became interested in going back into acting. The marriage suffered a strain when Hungarian-born British film director Alexander Korda signed her to a film contract. In 1935, when Korda was making a movie, she met English actor Lawrence Olivier who congratulated her on a stage role in *The Mask of Virtue*.

He was smitten with her. There could be nothing lovelier than her smile and looks. As his eyes took in the proud bearing of her figure, he must have thought her the very essence of beauty. Although both were married, they became lovers. Olivier recommended her as a tryout for the role of Scarlett O'Hara in David O. Selznick's upcoming *Gone with the Wind*. To increase patronage for that expensive movie, Selznick set out a world-wide contest for the best actress to play that role and Leigh won. She earned an Oscar for Best Actress in that movie.

She also played Ophelia to Olivier's *Hamlet* in an Old Vic production. But, shortly before going onstage one night, Leigh began screaming at Olivier for no apparent reason. She was calmed down by him and played the role but had no recollection of that event. He witnessed more strange behavior when they chose to live together despite both spouses refusing to divorce for some time. She developed a reputation with the film crew for being rude, unreasonable, and difficult.

Olivier was trying to become known in America so acted in the 1939 *Wuthering Heights*. She supported his efforts when he began to work on that movie. But she was so hyperactive that she could not sleep. She went for extremely long hours with little sleep, forgot her lines, and became quite ill. In the early 1950s, she saw psychoanalysts, but therapy did not seem productive for her. She went from one to another including Ralph Greenson and Laurence Kubie, both of whom were analysts who saw many celebrities. Kubie warned Olivier that her mood swings could become explosive and destroy relationships and her career.

Vivien preferred the stage to the screen but was a ravishing beauty. Directors wanted to use close-ups on the large screen. She could be very charming and almost weave a spell over someone because she was such a good actress. She once questioned whether her beauty made her more self-conscious and unsure of herself, thinking that only her appearance was valuable.

However, she began to be sexually indiscriminate and would confess her sins to Lawrence. He tried to help and loved her until the end of his life, according to numerous sources. She and Olivier finally parted ways due to her strange behavior and infidelities, causing him to say that she was not the person he married.

She played her role as an aging beauty in *Streetcar Named Desire* so well that she earned her second Academy Award for best actress. While co-star Marlon Brando played his role in that movie to great acclaim, a mentally ill actress playing a mentally ill woman of great beauty was the ultimate winner. She had played it on the stage and won the hearts of her audience. Her role in the movie remains one of the best portrayals ever seen by most reviewers. Some of her lines from movies can be pictured by readers because she acted them so very well.

As Blanche DuBois in Tennessee William's *A Streetcar Named Desire,* she said the devastating line that was so similar to her own life as she is taken away to a psychiatric hospital by a kindly man: "Whoever you are, I have always depended on the kindness of strangers."

Two of her unforgettable lines from *Gone with the Wind* were: "I can't think about that right now. If I do, I'll go crazy. I'll think about that tomorrow." "After all... tomorrow is another day."

She was found to have a manic-depressive (bipolar) illness in which she hallucinated and was driven to action day and night, followed by serious depression. It may have first appeared in 1937, but a miscarriage in 1944 seemed to trigger this major illness. It was best treated by medicine because the patient is unable, unwilling, and unhappy talking about anything except whatever momentary thought passes through her head.

It seemed nothing helped her, so a last resort was chosen. She was hospitalized and packed in ice as well as having electroshock therapy. Those treatments even left burn marks on her head. That treatment was in addition to treatment with Isoniazid for tuberculosis which spread to both lungs in May 1967. Such treatment causes much memory loss, and her career was fading quickly.[1]

After the divorce from Laurence Olivier, he married actress Joan Plowright. Vivien had a partner, Canadian-born British actor John Merivale, from 1960 until her death in 1967. He left the evening of July 7, 1967, to play a role on stage and returned home and got in bed. But he awoke later and found her on the floor. She had apparently attempted to walk to the bathroom and as her lungs filled with liquid from tuberculosis, she collapsed and suffocated.

Merivale called Olivier and they made the funeral arrangements together. The final tribute was read by actor Sir John Gielgud. Selections from her movies were shown to those at the funeral.

Note

1. https://truthaboutect.org/electroshock-runins-creativity-lives/
   https://vivienleigh.wordpress.com/2009/07/29/vivien-leigh-a-star-that-fell-victim-to-psychiatric-misdiagnosis-violent-treatment/

Oscar Levant

Oscar Levant (1906-1972) was a jazz pianist who was a close friend of George Gershwin. He was the son of Russian Jews who owned a jewelry store. His father demanded that his sons play songs exactly as he ordered. Levant rebelled against him as he later came to do against all authority figures in later life. His father died when he was 15, and Oscar left school for New York where he found musical work in nightclubs and speakeasies during the Prohibition era. He trained with excellent pianists and was expected to compose and play music of his own.

About 1925, he met George Gershwin and gradually became his sidekick and interpreter. In his autobiography, *The Memoirs of an Amnesiac,* published in 1965, on page 58, he described how George Raft, who was a professional dancer before becoming an actor, George Gershwin, and Levant were messing around one day. Raft did an amazingly fast Charleston dance to "Sweet Georgia Brown" which had just come out that year, and he bet Oscar that he could not play that jolting passage hitting all the notes. Raft lost the bet as Levant beat out the keys on the piano.

Sometimes Gershwin found it too strenuous to play all his songs himself and asked Oscar to play them. Gershwin apparently confided to some that he thought Oscar could play his songs better than he could.[1]

George Gershwin had a brain tumor that began to destroy his life. Levant played for him during his confusion when he could not appear. After Gershwin's death in 1937, Levant continued performances where he kept Gershwin's music alive, as well as playing works by other famous musicians.

Levant has been in many movies such as 1945 *Rhapsody in Blue*, 1948 *You Were Meant for Me*, 1949 *The Barkleys of Broadway*, 1951 *An American in Paris*, 1953 *The Band Wagon*, and 1955 *The Cobweb*. He was a quick-witted savant of music and became popular not only as a deft pianist but as a comedian and on radio quiz shows such as the 1938-1947 *Information Please,* and NBC's *Kraft Music Hall*.

Some of his acidic comments were "I knew Doris Day before she was a virgin," "I think a lot of Leonard Bernstein but not as much as he does," and "Now that Marilyn Monroe is kosher (when she married Jewish playwright Arthur Miller), Arthur Miller can eat her."

Levant was pictured in movies and elsewhere as always smoking a cigarette, drinking coffee, and unable to sleep. As the years went by, he continued to play the piano but wore himself down. He suffered a heart attack in 1950 and developed an addiction to his pain medicine, the opiate Demerol.

There is one report that Elizabeth Taylor and Montgomery Clift, who became close friends filming *A Place in the Sun*, used to drop by Levant's Beverly Hills home while they were working on the movie *Raintree County*. Oscar would play some Gershwin tunes and they would all use drugs.

Clift and Taylor had begun using marijuana with actor Peter Lawford and his son. Taylor had a birth defect in her spine and was often shot up with drugs like Novocain, hydrocortisone, Demerol, and Meticorten, a steroid used for inflammation. She was married to English actor Michael Wilding, but both were having affairs and drinking alcohol heavily.

Shortly before they divorced, on May 12, 1956, the Wildings threw a party where Clift was a guest. He drove away that night during a fog and crashed into a pole down the street. Hearing this, Elizabeth ran to the wreck, got to him through the broken back seat. She saved his life when his teeth became embedded in his tongue strangling him. She pulled his teeth out of his tongue and stopped photographers from photographing him.[2]

Back to Levant, his nerves and never-ending stage fright, demanding tour schedule, poor health, and descent into drug abuse just about ended his careerby 1955. He sought help first seeing psychoanalyst Ralph Greenson. Levant seemed no longer disposed to analysis. He had no taste for it. In addition, he was not a suitable candidate for psychoanalysis because of his drug abuse, so Ralph Greenson referred him to a psychiatrist who might manage his medicines.

Greenson loved to treat celebrities, but he expected them to be grateful to him and listen to his advice. It was not in Levant's nature to be grateful, or to admire and follow the advice of authority figures. He was disinclined to look within himself and discover why he had such feelings, and simply removed himself from emotions through drugs.

As his drug abuse grew, he required more containment so he could not get to the substances he abused. He finally checked himself in at Mt. Sinai Hospital. From there, he was given a four-hour furlough from his psychiatric unit to appear on television on various shows such as Jack Paar and *The Tonight Show* where his caustic wit was on display for audiences. Jack Paar used to close his show by saying, "Good night, Oscar Levant, wherever you are."

One of his doctors, George Wayne, M.D., even came on Oscar Levant's television show as a guest while Levant talked openly about his psychological problems. Poor Oscar had taken the breath away from audiences by his piano performances and his clever cynical utterances. Toward the end, he was an unhappy man who tried to keep people laughing.

From 1958 to 1960, Los Angeles TV studio KCOP ran *The Oscar Levant Show*, co-hosted by Oscar's wife, June, who sat beside him at a desk as they interviewed a few guests, and he played piano. His TV producer, Al Burton, would regularly check Levant out of the psychiatric unit at Mt. Sinai for 90 minutes of live TV, and then sign him back into the hospital.

Levant first married actress Barbara Woodell in 1932 and they divorced the following year. He later married singer June Gale in 1939 and remained married despite turmoil until his death. What a wonderful dispensation it is of Nature that every man, however superficially unattractive, should be some woman's choice.

He had three daughters. He wrote three autobiographies, 1940 *A Smattering of Ignorance,* 1965 *The Memoirs of an Amnesiac,* and 1968 *The Unimportance of Being Oscar.*

On August 13, 1972, soon to become actress Candice Bergen who was then a photojournalist, interviewed Levant and took a picture of him for her story. He asked her to return the next day for more information and photographs. She came back on August 14, 1972. When she rang the doorbell, Oscar's wife called him to come out from his bedroom. When he didn't answer, she went in and found him dead.[3]

In April 2021, the play *Good Night, Oscar*, by Doug Wright opened on Broadway at the Belasco Theater. Sean Hayes played Levant in a show about true events when he was allowed to leave the hospital for his media interviews.[4]

Notes

1. Caleb Taylor Boyd, *Oscar Levant: Pianist, Gershwinite, Middlebrow Media Star*, a dissertation published in 2020. https://openscholarship-wustl.edu/art_sci_edds/2169
2. Lisa's History Room: Michael Wilding: "How Liz Taylor Saved Monty Clift's Life" https://lisawallerrogers.com/tag/michael-wilding/
3. *Knock Wood* by Candace Bergen described this occurrence.
4. https://www.encyclopedia.com/history/encyclopedias-almanacs-transcripts-and-maps/oscar-levant

Peter Lorre

Peter Lorre was born Laszlo Lowenstein (1904-1964) in a Hungarian city which is now in Slovakia. His parents were German-speaking Jews, and his father was a lieutenant in the Austrian Army Reserve and bookkeeper at a local textile mill. His mother died when he was four. His father married his wife's best friend, but Peter never got along with her. He was alone a great deal. Solitude gives birth to the original in us.

His family moved to Vienna in 1913 when he was nine, and his father served in WWI. His loneliness set him to daydreaming as he imagined himself in settings with other people.

Lorre began acting on stage in Vienna at age 17. He moved on with fellow actors to Berlin in the 1920s. He was cast by director Fritz Lang as a child killer in the 1931 movie *M*. That unusual movie was about a man who whistled music just before he would kill a child. He whistled the haunting melody from Edvard Grieg's "In the Hall of the Mountain King" from the *Peer Gynt Suite*. Lorre couldn't whistle so director Lang whistled the tune for him in the movie.

The title came from someone thinking he was a murderer and writing M in white on back of his black coat. In one scene, he said in German, "I am better than the police." That coat with M, however, led people through a long chase and his capture. The movie was troubling and evocative, and established the talent of Lorre and director Lang.

In 1933, Lorre moved to London where Alfred Hitchcock's associate producer noticed him while making the 1934 film *The Man Who Knew Too Much*. After being selected to star in that movie, he gradually learned

English and moved to the United States with his first wife, Russian actress Celia Lovsky. They divorced in 1945 and he married Viennese actress Kaaren Vern that same year. They divorced in 1950, and he married publicist Anne Marie Brenning in 1954 who was with him until his death in 1964.

Peter and Anne had one child, daughter Catharine. She was kidnapped by Angelo Buono and Kenneth Bianchi who were known as the Hillside Strangler, because the press initially thought the murders were committed by one person. The two men terrorized Los Angeles for a five-month period beginning in October 1977 until the murders suddenly stopped in February of 1978.

The killers often posed as policemen to abduct their victims. On a night in 1977, they stopped Catharine Lorre, intending to kill her in the same gruesome manner as the other victims. But it turned out they were movie fans and learned she was Peter Lorre's daughter. They liked him because he played a serial killer in *M*. They released 25-year-old Catharine, even though it was thirteen years after her father had died. She never realized how close she had come to a brutal death until they were captured, and she saw their photographs. In later interviews she said she never felt threatened by the pair.[1]

Lorre was in movies such as 1935 *Mad Love*, 1935 *Crime and Punishment*, and 1936 *Secret Agent*. He was in several *Mr. Moto* movies playing a Japanese detective/spy and starred in *The Hunchback of Notre Dame*. He became frustrated with broken promises by Fox studios about better roles and ended his contract with them.

He became a naturalized citizen of the U.S. in 1941 and director John Huston cast him in *The Maltese*

Falcon. He enjoyed the company of Humphrey Bogart, Sydney Greenstreet and Claude Rains in movies such as *Casablanca, Background to Danger,* and *Passage to Marseilles,* etc. He returned to comedy with 1944 *Arsenic and Old Lace* starring Cary Grant. Here are some lines with Marian Marsh from 1935 *Crime and Punishment*.

> Lorre: I wonder how many poor devils have found an answer to their questions down there. If only the dead could come back.
> Marsh: They can! Remember the raising of Lazarus?
> Lorre: Are you happy to have your Bible back?
> Marsh: Would you like me to read you the raising of Lazarus?
> Lorre: I can't understand you. How can you continue living like this?
> Marsh: I believe in God.
> Lorre: What have you or I to hope for out of life?
> Marsh: Don't take away my faith. I need it.
> Lorre: Don't take away my unbelief. I need that.

He appeared before the House Un-American Activities Committee (HUAC) in 1947, having sympathized with John Huston and others in the short-lived Committee for the First Amendment. In 1949, he filed for bankruptcy. In 1950, he made a movie in West Germany which he had written, directed, and starred but it did not do well at the box office.

He returned to the U.S. where he played in a variety of movies and TV adaptations. In his last years, he worked with Roger Corman on low budget films including 1962 *Tales of Terror* with Vincent Price and Basil Rathbone, and 1963 *The Raven* with Price, Boris Karloff, and Jack Nicholson.

He suffered from gallbladder ailments and became addicted to morphine that the doctor prescribed. He struggled with his weight gain and career disappointments and died of a stroke in 1964. Vincent Price read his eulogy at the funeral. Actor Price had made his last five movies with Lorre and called his death a "tragedy." Price said, "Peter was the most inventive actor I've ever known. He was a great scholar, an accomplished dramatic actor, and a masterful comedian."

We shall never know exactly what Peter Lorre discussed with Dr. Ralph Greenson, but they had met earlier in Vienna, Austria. The troubled life of Peter Lorre and his heroin addiction suggest that this man and his analyst had much to work on during his time in therapy. Unlike most heroin users, Lorre managed to keep some control over his use and could handle therapy.

Greenson spoke of Lorre in a conversation with Richard Lemon, who wrote "Psychiatry, the Uncertain Science" for the *Saturday Evening Post* on August 10, 1968. Lemon and Greenson discussed how many laymen assume that psychiatrists have x-ray vision which enables them to read people's minds. Greenson said he had just such an example: "When I first practiced in Los Angeles, I went to Twentieth Century Fox to have lunch with a good friend of mine, Peter Lorre, whom I had known from Vienna. Wallace Beery was with us. Wallace Beery looked at me and then looked away and ate and ate and ate, and he finally said, 'Doc, what am I thinking?'"

Note

1. https://www.grunge.com/483987/how-peter-lorres-daughter-was-nearly-a-victim-of-the-hillside-strangler/

Vincente Minelli

Vincente Minnelli was born Lester Minelli (1903-1986) in Chicago from a French-Canadian actress and her husband, who was the musical conductor of Minnelli Brothers' Tent Theater. They traveled about doing shows where his mother appeared on stage. Early in his life, Vincente was living as a gay man working as a window dresser and photographer in Chicago.

He began work with a movie theater chain and became employed at the Radio City Music Hall as set designer and stage director, as well as color consultant of the Rainbow Room. The Rainbow Room was financed by the Rockefellers as a two-story nightclub atop the RCA building.

Vincente soon directed a musical revue in 1935 starring Beatrice Lillie, Ethel Waters, and Eleanor Powell. He went on to work on *The Ziegfeld Follies of 1936 and* was offered a job at MGM in 1940. He directed films such as 1943 *Cabin in the Sky*, 1943 *I Dood It*, and 1944 *Meet Me in St. Louis* where he fell in love with the film's young star Judy Garland.

His puzzling lifestyle was bisexual as he fashioned himself as a bohemian dandy surrounded by people like George and Ira Gershwin and satirical author Dorothy Parker. He ran into Garland, who had slept around with Frank Sinatra and others. She became jealous believing that Minnelli loved co-star, Gene Kelly, during the making of 1948 *The Pirate*.

Vincente struggled with masculinity issues when he directed 1956 *Tea and Sympathy*, 1957 *Designing Woman*, and 1960 *Home from the Hill*. He always suffered from being effeminate and sought help from psychoanalyst Ralph

Greenson. Minnelli was so private about his love life that he omitted it from his 1974 memoir, *I Remember It Well*.[1]

His relationship with Judy Garland led to marriage in 1945 and they had Liza Minnelli who grew up to become an Academy Award-winning actress and singer. The Minnelli household had a father, mother, and child who won Oscars. Minelli also directed Judy Garland in *The Big Clock* with Robert Walker and *The Pirate* with Gene Kelly.

Judy Garland's movie career took off big-time when she appeared in *The Wizard of Oz* singing her signature song, "Somewhere Over the Rainbow." However, she first appeared as a 13-year-old with her two sisters in a short 19-minute MGM film called *La Fiesta de Santa Barbara* which can be seen on the Internet. Others in that little movie are Andy Devine, Buster Keaton, Warner Baxter, Ida Lupino, Gilbert Roland, Robert Taylor, Harpo Marx, Gary Cooper, and Leo Carillo.

The Garland sisters sang "La Cucaracha" which translated means soldiers called cockroaches do not want to march anymore because they do not have marijuana to smoke. Did little Judy know what they were singing about? The Spanish words are these: La cucaracha, la cucaracha, ya no puede caminar, porque no tiene, porque la falta, marijuana que fumar.

Back to Judy's husband, Vincente Minnelli directed musicals such as 1951 *An American in Paris*, 1954 *Brigadoon*, 1955 *Kismet*, and 1958 *Gigi*, as well as melodramatic movies. His marriage to Judy Garland ended in 1951, whereafter he married Georgette Magnani 1954-1958, Danica de Gigante 1962-1971, and Margaretta Lee Anders from 1980 until his death from emphysema, pneumonia, and Alzheimer's disease.

Judy Garland had been in treatment with Dr. Herbert Kupper who ran a psychoanalyst group in Los Angeles. He had been told that Garland was a pill popper and might fall into the wrong hands of doctors who coould offer relief through pills. She was about to be cast in the 1947 musical *Easter Parade* with songs by Irving Berlin and co-stars such as Fred Astaire. Kupper was hired to help the movie studio keep Garland productive and was opposed to her seeing another analyst like Dr. Ralph Greenson who gave medicines that might be overused.

When Kupper heard that Minnelli wanted Garland to see Greenson, he had Minnelli removed from the MGM musical. Vincente was humiliated and put himself into more sessions with Greenson. *Easter Parade* became the highest-grossing musical movie.

We all know that Judy Garland died of an overdose of Seconal sleeping pills. Her mother had begun her on pills to keep her weight down and her working hours up. She had married bandleader David Rose from 1941-44, Vincente Minelli 1945-51, Sid Luft 1952-55, actor Mark Herron 1965-69, and young musician Mickey Dean in 1969.

She died at age 47 on June 22, 1947. Co-star James Mason in *A Star Is Born* gave the eulogy at her funeral. She spent her last days doing shows to pay off IRS debts. Daughter Liza asked Frank Sinatra to help pay off her last debts after Judy's death and he did so.[2]

Minnelli's last movie, 1976 *A Matter of Time,* was his attempt to bring together parents, children, and old movie memories. It starred his daughter Liza, Ingrid Bergman and her daughter Isabella Rossellini, Jean Pierre Aumont's daughter Tina Aumont, and Charles Boyer. After all, Boyer and Bergman had so enjoyed their earlier collaborations, that their brief contact was quite sentimental. Sadly, this movie was not popular and was probably more satisfying to those in it than it was to audiences.

Boyer's wife was diagnosed with terminal cancer the following year, and this was his last movie. He committed suicide the day after she died on August 28, 1978. Vincente Minnelli's legacy was the many great films he produced and the many stars who won Oscars in his pictures.

Notes

1. https://www.advocate.com/arts-entertainment/film/2009/05/15/real-vincente-minnelli?
2. "The Tragic Final Months of Judy Garland's Life" by Lauren Hubbard, *Town & Country Magazine,* September 29, 2019.

Marilyn Monroe

Marilyn Monroe was born to Norma Jeane Mortenson (1926-1962) and a co-worker in Los Angeles, California. Marilyn's mother developed schizophrenia and was hospitalized. Marilyn spent most of her childhood in many foster homes and an orphanage. She escaped that at age 16 by marrying James Dougherty and dropping out of high school. She worked in a factory where a photographer took pictures of her for pin-up girl calendars and centerfolds. Her husband was in the Merchant Marines and shipped out to the Pacific and they divorced when he returned and found her busy having a career as a starlet.

At 20, she began to appear in small movie parts and did modeling part time. There was a scandal when she posed nude for a calendar in 1949, but it made her even more famous.

After some roles in *All About Eve* and *Asphalt Jungle* in 1950, she was featured in the Army newspaper *Stars and Stripes* as Miss Cheesecake of 1951.

She had some short relationships with men such as actors Yul Brynner and Peter Lawford and then met New York Yankees baseball star Joe DiMaggio in 1952. Her marriage with DiMaggio was short-lived from 1954-1955. He wanted to get her away from people he thought were bad for her. He did not want her to flaunt herself about. She signed a contract to do *The Seven-Year Itch* and left him, but they remained friends.

She took acting classes by Michael Chekhov and others. She then began a Fox contract by playing roles as a dumb blonde. She wanted to develop more skills so worked with acting coach Paula Strasberg. That irritated directors because she asked for so many re-takes at Paula's direction. Unfortunately, she began to use barbiturates, amphetamines, and alcohol for her anxiety and insomnia so that she forgot her lines and became severely addicted.

In 1956, she met and married author Arthur Miller. In 1957, she starred with Laurence Olivier in *The Prince and the Showgirl*. She starred with Tony Curtis and Jack Lemmon in *Some Like It Hot* in 1958, where she made life miserable for the cast by her tardiness and forgetfulness. She was given supposedly cute lines in that movie such as: "Real diamonds. They must be worth their weight in gold."

She made the musical comedy *Let's Make Love* with Yves Montand in 1960 which did not fare well at the box office. The Frenchman was probably amused by her comment in *Gentlemen Prefer Blondes:* "Is this the way to Europe, France?" as if she didn't know any geography.

She wanted Miller to write a movie to show her acting talent, so he wrote 1961*The Misfits*. He tended to write new lines during production, but she had trouble remembering them. Their marriage collapsed during filming, and they obtained a Mexican divorce in January 1961 just before the movie came out.

She was in treatment with Ralph Greenson for several years. He found her unable to do typical psychoanalysis where she would set her own goals of what kind of person she wanted to be and what she wanted to work on. She needed help with her divorce, so Ralph recommended Milton Alexander Rudin who had married Greenson's sister. Rudin had arranged Frank Sinatra's divorce from Mia Farrow. He also arranged the purchase of a house near Dr. Greenson during the last months of Marilyn's life. The analyst asked friend Eunice Murray to be her housekeeper and helpmate and keep him informed of any problems.

Dr. Greenson felt he should show her what a family was like, so in addition to therapy, he invited her for meals with his family, who became sort of relatives for her. She went to London for some filming, and he arranged for her to see Anna Freud, Sigmund's daughter who did child analysis. Because Monroe was so well paid, she gave large donations to Miss Freud to perpetuate treatment in her father's name for others. Greenson and Freud exchanged many letters about Marilyn Monroe and her difficulties. Greenson and her physician gave her medicines for sleep and anxiety.

President John Kennedy was introduced to Marilyn Monroe in February of 1962 when his brother-in-law, British actor Peter Lawford, invited her to a dinner party in New York being held to honor JFK. Monroe arrived over an hour late. The President took her arm, and they went to the table. He apparently asked for her phone number and called her the next day, saying that he would be in Palm Springs on March 24.[1]

Philip Watson, a former Los Angeles County assessor, was present when Monroe met Kennedy on March 24th at Bing Crosby's Spanish-style house in Palm Springs. Watson said that Monroe was wearing a kind of robe so that they were obviously intimate that night. Kennedy's friend, Florida Democratic Senator George Smathers, and a Secret Service agent later stated that they knew about the weekend.

The weekend in Palm Springs developed into an obsession for Monroe, who desperately wanted to see Kennedy again. Her publicist Rupert Allan described her as being "fixated on the President."[2,3]

For his part, President Kennedy sent Bing Crosby a note dated April 2, 1962, thanking him. He wrote: "Dear Bing, You will never know how much I enjoyed my weekend at your ranch. I can truthfully say that my stay there was one of the most pleasant and restful that I have had for a long time. I, therefore, want to thank you for making this possible."[4]

Marilyn Monroe made a disturbing phone call to President Kennedy's private line which Jacqueline Kennedy answered. Marilyn asked Jackie Kennedy if she could speak to JFK.[5] We can assume that the First Lady discussed this with the President. While we do not know the details of their discussion, we can assume that the president did not want his paramour to create problems for him.

Monroe began to make another movie with Dean Martin called *Something's Got to Give* but became ill with various problems such as sinusitis. She did not appear for weeks but took a break to sing *"Happy Birthday"* to President John Kennedy on May 19, 1962, at Madison Square Garden in New York. She was worried about being able to sing well so Dr. Max Jacobson, who is described later, gave her an injection in her neck to relax her vocal cords. She sang to the President slurring her words slightly in a breathy sort of manner.

She apparently felt she was being tossed aside by the President and by many others such as her director and co-stars. She was also wrestling with a career that depended upon looks. She may not have been pleased with her gradual aging. She swam nude as they were preparing for that last movie, against the director's order. She wanted to please men by showing herself, in hopes of better acceptance based on her body. A movie has been made about her last movie that was never produced. It can be seen on YouTube at https://www.youtube.com/watch?v=wDKeZO9Pe50 and other sites.

It was impossible for her to recover her poise or tranquility. Everybody was mad at her, her body was changing, and she was dependent upon mind-altering drugs. Her time had come to make an exit.

On August 4, 1962, Eunice Murray spent the night in Monroe's house and awoke at 3 a.m. seeing a light from under her bedroom door. She knocked and tried the door, but it was locked. She called Dr. Greenson, and he came over quickly. Frustrated with the locked door, he went outside and looked through a window where he saw her body on the bed. So, he broke the window to enter. He found her dead with several empty medicine bottles nearby. She had a telephone in her hand and had called Peter Lawford but could not speak clearly. He believed she said something about him being a nice guy. Deputy coroner Thomas Noguchi classified her death as a probable suicide.

A toxicology report showed acute barbiturate poisoning with 8 mg% chloral hydrate and 4.5 mg% pentobarbital (Nembutal) in her blood and 13 mg% pentobarbital in her liver, several times the lethal limit.

On August 5, 1962, authorities at Monroe's house did not know what to do or who to call, as Monroe had no family. They called DiMaggio who stepped in and orchestrated his ex-wife's funeral assisted by her half-sister Berniece Baker Miracle. DiMaggio barred the public and almost all the Hollywood glitterati, producers, directors, and actors from the funeral.[6]

He had the body attired in a favorite Pucci dress, had her movie hairdresser arrange her looks, and spent the night beside the casket in the Chapel of Palms. He invited around thirty to attend. Her acting teachers, her maid Eunice Murray, her driver and masseur, her lawyer Mickey Rudin, and her psychiatrist, Dr. Greenson and his family. Her first husband, James Dougherty and Arthur Miller chose not to attend.

The strains of "Somewhere Over the Rainbow," one of Marilyn's favorite songs, echoed through the chapel. Those present recited the 23rd psalm and a tearful Lee Strasberg delivered the eulogy. He ended with "I cannot say goodbye. Marilyn never liked good-byes, but in that peculiar way she had of turning things around so that they face reality—I will say *au revoir*. For the country to which she has gone, we must all someday visit."

Tearful Joe DiMaggio stood over the casket, kissed her for the last time, placed three roses in her hand and whispered, "I love you." Twice a week for the next twenty years, DiMaggio visited her grave and left flowers.[7]

Marilyn left a quarter of her large estate to her first psychoanalyst Marianne Kris. Most of the rest of her fortune went to her acting coach Lee Strasberg and was later controlled by his relatives.

When Dr. Kris died in 1980, her share was passed on to the Anna Freud Centre, which has since thrived on the generosity and the income generated by license deals connected with Monroe. It provides support to children, working with youngsters who suffer from mental illness or are in emotional distress. Her funds helped children from 1962 to 2010. The Anna Freud Centre began to run short of funds and published a request in 2010 for donations to supplement it.[8]

Marilyn Monroe would probably have been happy to know that her generous funds have helped so many children who could, as a result of her generosity, have a better life. She was unable to deliver any children because of miscarriages but she has delivered them in this special way.

She asked so many people like husbands, directors, doctors, and lovers questions that could be translated as "Why hast thou forsaken me?" Joe Dimaggio did not.

Notes

1. "Sinatra's High Hopes Dashed by JFK"—Bing Crosby Internet Museum stevenlewis.info/Crosby/kennedy.htm
2. potus-geeks.livejournal.com/1112073.html
3. https://www.irishcentral.com/bing-crosby-mansion-jfk-marilyn-monroe
4. https://www.jfklibrary.org/asset-viewer/archives/JFKPOF/107/JFKPOF-107-018
5. https://www.dailymail.co.uk/news/article-12311063/Marilyn-Monroe-disturbing-phone-call-asking-Jackie-Kennedy-spek-JFK.html
6. https://www.pbs.org/wgbh/americanexperience/features/dimaggio-joe-directs-marilyns-funeral/
7. https://www.qcc.cuny.edu/socialsciences/ppecorino/SS680/Funeral_Marilyn_Monroe.html
8. themarilynmonroecollection.com/anna-freud-centre-funded-by-marilyn-monroe-suffers-financial-losses/

Frank Sinatra

Francis Albert Sinatra (1915-1998) was born to Italian immigrants living in New Jersey who ran a tavern. His father, Antonino "Marty" Sinatra, was a bantam weight boxer who used the name Marty O'Brien. His mother was a midwife. At birth, he had to be delivered by forceps which caused scarring to his left cheek, neck, and ear, and perforated his eardrum which resulted in him being unsuitable for military service. His mastoid bone was operated on, resulting in scarring on his neck and cystic acne that scarred his face and neck.

As he grew up around his parent's tavern, he began to sing songs on a player piano for spare change. He never learned to read music but played and sang by ear. He was influenced by Bing Crosby, Rudy Vallee, and Russ Colombo, and began to perform with his own group for school dances. He was expelled from high school for rowdiness. He worked as a delivery boy for newspapers and as a riveter for the shipyard. He continued to entertain and sing for his supper or for cigarettes.

His group performed on the Major Bowes Amateur Hour, gaining a contract to perform on stage and radio across the U.S. He became a singing waiter in 1938, worked in a roadhouse, and performed with a group during the Dance Parade show. He joined the Harry James group and began to record songs. He went over to the Tommy Dorsey band, and the skinny kid with big ears gradually gained popularity. By 1940, he was known for several song successes.

As men were drafted for WWII, he was not and became a bobby-sox idol as a singer. He entertained troops in the USO and Sinatra fan clubs sprang up everywhere. He sometimes sang with the popular Andrews sisters on the radio.

From 1945-46, he starred in four movies. He played the role of a priest in *The Miracle of the Bells*, but after negative publicity about Mafia connections, he decided to donate $100,000 to the Catholic church.

Gradually, his career was going downhill, and record sales diminished. He had married Nancy Barbato whom he met doing lifeguard duty in 1939, and they had three children. He divorced Nancy in 1951 because he fell in love with actress Ava Gardner. He married Gardner from 1951 to 1957 and their public and private fights made notable news headlines. Their tempestuous relationship caused him to be suicidal and he tried to kill himself with gas and sleeping pills. His agent, who was married to Ralph Greenson's sister, recommended that Frank see Dr. Greenson.

He took up therapy with Greenson for his depression over the separation from Gardner, but his movie career kept him moving about. He was booked in Las Vegas where he became a regular entertainer with the Rat Pack which included Dean Martin, Sammy Davis Jr., Jack Warden, Joey Bishop, Peter Lawford, and various others. His acting revived his career, especially when he won an Academy award for his part in *From Here to Eternity* released in 1953. Here are some of his lines in that movie:

Sinatra: I just hate to see a good guy get it in the gut.

Warden: You better get used to it, kid. You'll probably see a lot of it before you die.

Clift: You've been hoggin' the Whiskey, Angelo.

Sinatra: Not me buddy. It's that Sandra, she's a nice girl, but she drinks like a fish! Let's go to a phone booth or something, huh? Where I will unveil a fifth of whiskey, I have hidden here under my loose, flowing sports shirt.

Frank Sinatra knew Peter Lawford, President John Kennedy's in-law, so he supported the President. He also played and sang for other presidents and notable figures.

As time passed, his voice began to change, and he collapsed once during a stage presentation. He tried to continue performing but had hearing problems by this time as well. He had a brief affair with Marilyn Monroe but became terribly upset with Ralph Greenson when he saw the dismal condition of the actress. Sinatra saw syringes and medicines falling out of her purse, apparently given to her by a variety of her physicians. Old Blue Eyes did not want to be associated with her anymore. He realized she was addicted and had serious mental deterioration.

Frank Sinatra went on to marry young actress Mia Farrow, some 29 years younger than himself. She was the daughter of actress Maureen O'Sullivan, who had played the love interest of Tarzan in early movies. Sinatra and Farrow's brief marriage from 1966 to 1968 was followed by his long marriage to Barbara Marx. By the time he met Barbara, Frank had roved about living this place and that, and he sought a fresh and stable scene with a lovemate.

Barbara had been married to Zeppo Marx, the handsome young Marx brother. Frank gradually became debilitated due to his long history of smoking and drinking and died of a heart attack. After prolonged caretaking by Barbara, he was mourned by his wife and children when he died at age 83. Thousands turned out for his funeral and a skywriter sketched a white heart on the blue sky.[1]

Note

1. Petkov, Steven; Mustazza, Leonard (1995). *The Frank Sinatra Reader.* Oxford University Press. ISBN 978-0-19-509531-9.

Inger Stevens

Inger Stevens was born Ingrid Stensland (1934-1970) in Stockholm, Sweden. Her mother left the family for another man when Inger was six years old. Her father came to America on a Fulbright scholarship leaving Inger and her brother with a maid and later an aunt.

Upon earning a Ph.D., he sent for his children. Inger was unhappy in that Kansas home where her father taught college and disliked his new wife. She ran away and got into a burlesque theater as a dancer. Her father brought her home, and she finally graduated high school. She then left for New York where she studied acting under Lee Strasburg while working as a chorus girl.

She married Anthony Soglio (1955-58) who acted as her agent and got her into television and movies. She starred in *Man of Fire* with Bing Crosby and fell in love with him. Their affair was known to many and after he married Lee Grant, she was heartbroken.

She went on to star in the 1959 Harry Belafonte movie *The World, the Flesh, and the Devil*. She was reported to have had an affair with Belafonte, who was married to second wife Julie Robinson, during the filming. At the end of filming, he returned to his wife.

The desolate actress went to a New Year's Eve Party and on the morning of January 1, 1959, mixed Seconal (a barbiturate hypnotic) with alcohol and ammonia intending to die. She survived, with minor blood clots in both legs and temporary vision impairment in both eyes.

Belafonte's company, HarBel Productions, had Vice President Isaac (Ike) Jones, also a black man. He was the first African American producer of a major Hollywood film. That film was 1965 *A Man Called Adam* starring Sammy Davis Jr. and Louis Armstrong. Ike also managed Nat King Cole's production company. Ike and Inger became involved with each other and went to Tijuana, Mexico, to be married in the fall of 1961. Their marriage remained a secret because she feared it would wreck her career due to racial prejudice. Inger told only her brother. Their nine-year marriage was strained by long separations.

Two years before she died, she made *Firecreek* appearing with Henry Fonda and James Stewart. This movie dialogue demonstrated a woman who was trying to reform a man she cared about:

Stevens: "It's obvious you and your men are hired killers down from the northern range wars."
Fonda: "We work in the open. We eat and drink with the ranchers who hire us and are as much respected as anyone in the country."
Stevens: "Don't quibble any fine line with me, Mr. Larkin. You're as dishonest as any common road bandit."
Fonda: "I'm not ashamed of the part I play.... You tie me up pretty good, Evelyn."
Stevens: "Why fight against times changing? Why not join in changing them."
Fonda: "Then I'll be like all the rest. Today I'm one of the few. I lead. That's important to me."

She went to see Ralph Greenson to discuss some issues with men. Unfortunately, he used pharmaceuticals as a kind of parental support or comfort when he was unable to have regular contact with some patients. One of her letters to Dr. Greenson said the following:

> I live in a constant state of insecurity and crippling anxiety that I try to hide by appearing cold. People think I am aloof, but really, I am just scared. I often feel depressed. I come from a broken home, my marriage was a disaster, and I am constantly lonely... I don't want to die thinking all I've been doing is passing time, heading on down the road until I crawl off into my grave. I'd like to leave something behind me, to contribute to my generation's legacy, I'll do that through my work as an actress.[1]

She wanted to be something, to have some significance. She had tried to help people in mental health associations but that was so distant from her own person. Her loneliness and depression were not helped by someone who lived with her since she was apart from her husband. Perhaps Greenson's medicines for Inger Stevens were like those he gave to Marilyn Monroe. He wrote this about Monroe's medications:

> When I left for a five-week summer vacation, I felt it was indicated to leave her some medication which she might take when she felt depressed and agitated, i.e., rejected and tempted to act out. I prescribed a drug which is a quick-acting anti-depressant in combination with a sedative—Dexamyl... The administering of the pill was an attempt to give her something of me to swallow, to take in, so that she could overcome the sense of terrible emptiness that would depress and infuriate her.[2]

What he gave Stevens was twenty-five pills of Seconal and Tedral. The latter drug is an asthma and chronic obstructive pulmonary disease medicine that contained a kind of bronchodilator that made a person wakeful, so it was combined with phenobarbital to enhance sleep. Stevens washed those down with alcohol on April 30, 1970, at age 36.

She was found in an apartment she shared with Lola McNally. After her death, Ike Jones signed for the release of her body as her next of kin. Her $171,000 estate allowed him some money which he donated to mental health organizations which she had chaired and worked with. Perhaps she was filled with good intentions, but the darker side of human nature prevailed within her. Inger's brother verified that she had married Ike in Mexico and kept it a secret.[3]

Los Angeles county coroner Dr. Thomas Noguchi called her death a suicide by "acute barbiturate poisoning." William Patterson wrote *The Farmer's Daughter Remembered: The Biography of Actress Inger Stevens,* published by Xlibris, in 2000.

Notes

1. Greenson's public lectures in the book *On Loving, Hating, & Living Well,* International Universities, 1992.
2. Greenson's public lectures in the book *On Loving, Hating, & Living Well,* International Universities, 1992.
3. https://www.scandinaviastandard.com/what-ever-happened-to-inger-stevens/

CHAPTER FIVE
Max Jacobson, M.D.

Max Jacobson (1900-1979) was born of Jewish parents in Fordon, Poland, part of the German Empire at that time. He earned his medical degree from the Friedrich Wilhelm University of Berlin. His doctoral dissertation was "The Clinical Significance of Choline on High Blood Pressure." In medical school, he investigated the influence of insulin on blood. From 1925-1931, he worked under Professor August Bier studying how to transplant tissues and organs.

He developed some interest in the field of psychiatry and knew of Sigmund Freud, Carl Jung, and Alfred Adler who occasionally met and lectured in Berlin. However, talking therapy was not of interest to a man who considered himself a scientist. So, he began to experiment with pharmaceuticals and mind-altering drugs. He looked for ways to mix such drugs with vitamins, enzymes, animal placentas, and hormones to cure illnesses such as malnutrition or abuse of alcohol or tranquilizers. Germany was dealing with WWI soldiers who lost limbs and his injections of liquid methamphetamines with goat and sheep blood helped patients to withstand stress and get their mind off their difficulties.

In 1932, Hitler's anti-Jewish policies were a threat to Jewish professionals, so Jacobson escaped to Prague, Czechoslovakia, where he received recognition for the development of a new process of sterilization. That enabled him to soon immigrate to France in 1933 where he became an associate of the Louis Pasteur Institute in urology. There he studied sulfa drugs in the treatment of gonorrhea.

An interest in athletics gave Dr. Jacobson the incentive to evaluate amino acids for people in athletic training. He became the medical supervisor of the French Olympic ladies swimming and tennis teams. While in Paris, he developed a method of lung lavage for use in the treatment of tuberculosis and investigated surgical rehabilitation methods.

In 1936, Jacobson emigrated to the United States, establishing a practice in New York City. He was appointed Assistant Visiting Surgery at the New York City Cancer Institute in 1938, from which he soon resigned to devote more time to the fields of vitamins therapy and amino acids. He wrote many articles in medical journals and one of the earliest articles on geriatrics.

During WWII, he worked with the Office of War Information, broadcasting medical and health advice in foreign languages for the use of underground fighters in several Nazi-occupied countries. He was celebrated as a man who spoke many languages.

He became a draft board physician and conducted research for preventing nerve damage occurring in war trauma. The treatment he described in the *New York State Journal of Medicine* in an article published October 1, 1945, was the first to apply the action of amino acid-vitamin combinations.

He established a medical practice in New York. We do not know what became of a first wife, but he married Nina Hagen in 1946. She would die in 1964, possibly from using her husband's concoctions. His studies in vitamin therapy with hormones and enzymes using injections of organic substrates were often tried out on himself as well as his patients.

Together with Dr. Charles Ressler, he developed a quick cure for infectious hepatitis combining cortisone with broad spectrum antibiotics, eliminating months of bed confinement. That was described in his article published by the *New York State Journal of Medicine* on October 1, 1956. For some ten years, he centered attention on neuromuscular ailments such as multiple sclerosis, muscular dystrophy, and rheumatoid arthritis.

His methods consisted of injecting selective tissue enzymes, organic substrates, and vitamins into the body to replace diseases or old cellular material. He wanted to counteract the stresses of those who live and work under continual high pressure. In the beginning, to his credit he did not refuse treatment to anyone, regardless of a patient's business or financial status. That behavior began to change when he was so busy that he took only very important people as patients.

His work came to the attention of Claude Pepper, Chairman of a committee described in *Crime in America— Heroin Importation and Distribution Hearings before the Select Committee on Crimes* in June 1970. Jacobson was asked to testify, and he recommended that drug users should be given other drugs to keep them and their children from addiction.

By that time, his practice had grown as patients and celebrities began using his injections. Since many of his injections included amphetamines, patients became addicted to his treatments. He was called Miracle Max and Dr. Feelgood.[1]

Jacobson never really understood the fact that you may nurture others, but if you allow them to become dependent upon you, you're really hurting them, not helping them. He was known for his "miracle tissue regenerator" shots which consisted of amphetamines, animal hormones, bone marrow, enzymes, human placenta, steroids, and multivitamins. But the amphetamines made patients need more and more and more.

By the late 1960s, Jacobson's own behavior became strange as he worked 24-hour days, saw up to thirty patients per day, and his patient, former presidential photographer Mark Shaw, died at the age of 47 of "acute and chronic intravenous amphetamine poisoning." Max wanted to be needed by important people like movie stars, musicians, politicians, and especially President John Kennedy.

There was an original title for the movie *Casablanca* called *Everybody Comes to Ricks,* but some patients used the words *"Everybody Comes to Dr. Jacobson."*

Jacobson's staff admitted buying huge quantities of amphetamines to give many high-level doses. The Bureau of Narcotics and Dangerous Drugs seized Jacobsons' supply, and his medical license was revoked on April 25, 1975, by the New York State Board of Regents.

Among the charges of unprofessional conduct filed against Dr. Jacobson were illegal possession of amphetamines and the distribution of misbranded and mislabeled drugs. The charge of fraud alleged that the doctor illegally dispensed amphetamines to many people without performing a medical examination.

Dr. Jacobson tried to renew his license but met with denial. Life is like that. It does not permit you to arrange and order it as you will. He died on December 1, 1979, and he was buried next to his second wife, Nina.

We will now look closely at some of his patients to learn how he wanted to be their savior, but many of them needed to be saved from him.

Note

1. https:www.medicalbag.com/home/features/despicable-doctors/the-secret-service-gave-him-the-code-name-dr-feelgood/

Maria Callas

Maria Callas was born Maria Kalogeropoulos (1923-1977) in New York City to impoverished Greek parents. They returned to Greece during her childhood. Her natural beauty was hidden early because she was a chubby youngster. However, her extraordinary voice soon attracted attention and led to a career in classical opera. She received her musical education in Greece and developed her career in Italy. She had an incredibly wide-ranging voice and could do dramatic interpretations. However, she was extremely near-sighted, and was nearly blind on-stage in early life.

She was temperamental, endured struggles, scandals, and developed a bad reputation in some places. She was praised for her work in the operas of Donizetti, Bellini, Rossini, Verdi, Puccini, and even Wagner. Her bel canto technique and voice were so stupendous that she was hailed as "the divine one."

She met and married Giovanni Battista Meneghini, a wealthy industrialist some thirty years older than she in 1949, and he assumed control of her career. He, like her mother, stole from her funds over the years.

She was unlucky in love, unhappy in stopping others from living off her success and was not pleased with her looks. She had been very plump but lost half her body weight at age thirty, when she took a dangerous experimental drug in Switzerland in 1953. The weight loss changed her voice, some say for the better and some say for the worse. No longer could anybody say around her, "It ain't over till the fat lady sings."

Her depression and unhappiness took away her vitality. In New York, many talked about Dr. Max Jacobson. Since her experimental drug in 1953 was successful, she was willing to try his vitamin concoction in the mid-1950s. He promised her more energy and good spirits with his "liquid vitamins." He then injected her with vitamin B, amphetamine, and methamphetamine, called "speed" on the street. She gradually became addicted to the drugs.

Jacobson was like her Svengali, the man who seduced and hypnotized Trilby and made her into a famous singer. Jacobson kept supplying her and she tried to keep performing, but her work began to suffer. Audiences were more critical. It all became too much for her. She experienced a nervous breakdown in 1958 and was hospitalized for that and for her anorexic eating disorder.

In early 1959, she and her husband were invited for a cruise by shipping magnate Aristotle (called Ari) Onassis aboard his floating palace yacht. Another on board was former British Prime Minister Winston Churchill. Churchill sailed with Onassis eight times between 1958 and 1963, and one of his paintings hung in the yacht saloon. Callas was courted during that cruise by Onassis and at the end of their cruise, Marie asked her husband for a divorce which was granted in 1959.

She began a nine-year affair with Onassis and may have become pregnant but lost or aborted the child. Onassis was attracted by her celebrity status. For example, Callas and Giuseppe Di Stefano drove the audience wild at La Scala Opera House in Milan on May 28, 1955, when they sang *La Traviata*. However, Ari did not intend to marry her. Despite the Callas-Onassis affair, Aristotle invited Jacqueline Kennedy and her sister, Lee Radziwill, to sail with him. Both ladies had affairs with Onassis, but at different times.

Aristotle was a short man and both Maria Callas and wife Jacqueline Kennedy Onassis were much taller than he. Maria felt terrible when she learned of Onassis' wedding to the Kennedy widow. She had so wished to marry Aristotle, but Onassis had many goals, and a marriage with her was not among them.

Years earlier, Onassis had problems with the United States when he negotiated a deal to supply Saudi Arabian oil tankers. The American oil industry and the Saudi King had an agreement which he violated. Washington leaders learned of his deal and repossessed his tankers as they docked in America, seizing his profits. He pled guilty and paid $7 million, so the criminal charges against him were dropped.

When Onassis married Jacqueline Kennedy, he left Callas behind and she toured Europe with Giuseppe Di Stefano. After Onassis' marriage to Kennedy, Callas was forced go back to work. She attempted to find success in movies but that did not work out and she began to teach music and tour during the 1970s.

Maria and singing partner Giuseppe became lovers, but everlasting love was an unknown experience for her. Giuseppe wanted nothing more than wine, women, and song. Maria died of a heart attack alone in her Paris apartment on September 16, 1977, at age 53. The end of her life was almost like the operas she sang with a melodramatic finale.

Onassis and Jackie honeymooned on his exclusive island of Scorpios, Greece. There she said "I do" surrounded by family. Her children, John and Caroline, participated by holding candles during the ceremony. Jackie's sister, Lee Radziwill, was the matron of honor. Around forty guests witnessed the 45-minute ceremony.

Onassis later took Jackie to Athens. Here, Socrates held forth upon the nature of virtue and desire. But as Onassis gazed at the beauty of his young wife, he worshipped her. He was the perfect Aladdin, making her dreams come true. And some of his own dreams came true through this union, which could never have happened with Maria Callas.

The shipping magnate had evened the score with the Kennedys by this marriage after Robert Kennedy had accused him of corruption in the shipping industry. He helped himself in other ways. The Onassis' yacht "Christina" had hosted Grace Kelly's honeymoon to Prince Rainier III of Monaco, for an intimate wedding reception. He did that because his Monaco investments ran into trouble after WWII. After that Rainier wedding, Monaco was then a place to see and be seen and he had helped his own investments in that little principality.[1-4]

Notes

1. https://www.ranker.com/list/aristotle-onassis-marriage-of-grace-kelly/rachel-souerbry
2. https://www.brides.com/story/jackie-kennedy-aristotle-onassis-wedding-photos
3. https://www.theguardia.com/music/2021/apr/11/drugged-sexually-abused-swindled-maria-callas-tormented-life-revealed
4. https://www.phillips.com/churchill
   Sir Winston L.S. Churchill. "Painting as a Pastime," *The Strand Magazine,* December 21, p. 537.

Truman Capote

Truman Capote (1924-1984) was born in New Orleans to a salesman and his wife. His parents divorced when he was two and he was raised by relatives until he was eleven. Then his mother married a Spanish colonel who adopted Truman. He suffered from loneliness and tried to act up to gain attention. In later life, his dangerous acting up on drugs supplied by Max Jacobson led to shunning by others, and death by an overdose of some kind of drug.

At age 18, he became a copyboy in the art department of *The New Yorker* where he was fired two years later for making poet Robert Frost angry. He moved to Alabama where he was found, on examination for the Armed Services during WWII, to be "too neurotic." He tended to exhibit rather swishy mannerisms, undoubtedly intended to attract attention. Military authorities may have foreseen that he would need to follow orders without individual attention being paid.

In Alabama he was a friend and neighbor of Harper Lee who wrote *To Kill a Mockingbird* in 1960. Her father was a lawyer, and they occasionally went to some trials together. In fact, Truman claimed to be a character in that book.

He became a novelist, screenwriter, playwright, and actor. He authored many short stories, was extremely intelligent, and could create stories about characters with unusual habits. He was a keen observer of others and studied their dispositions and their manner of talking.

His most famous works are the novella *Breakfast at Tiffany's* and the crime novel *In Cold Blood* in 1966 about an actual murder of a Kansas farm family. It became a novel but was based on extensive research about the actual events.

Harper Lee helped him in his research for *In Cold Blood*. The novelist was often distracted but pulled himself together and began to write a new kind of book combining fiction and fact. He took his fountain pen and swung around to Harper, beguiled by her voice, each time she had a thought for him. He had a lot of courage on paper. Movies were made of both books and his search for fame was realized. Here are some lines from *In Cold Blood* and *Breakfast at Tiffany's*:

"I thought that Mr. Clutter was a very nice gentleman. I thought so right up to the moment that I cut his throat."

"There's got to be something wrong with us. To do what we did."

"Well, when I get it, the only thing that does any good is to jump in a cab and go to Tiffany's. Calms me down right away."

"I don't want to own anything until I find a place where me and things go together. I'm not sure where that is but I know what it is like. It's like Tiffany's."

He never did live like Harper Lee. He lived a decadent life, in gay cities patronized by high society. He never married and lived an openly homosexual life with men who were usually authors. There were connections with another gay author, Tennessee Williams, and the two men had a great deal of respect for each other.

In his later years, Capote's alcoholism, drug use, and cocaine addiction became a problem and required control and additional treatment. He was in and out of various rehabilitation hospitals and clinics.

He enjoyed using his imagination. Drug use invited him to experience things he would describe. He wrote about the treatments he received from Dr. Max Jacobson. He used these interesting words to describe the effects of the liquid vitamins:

> You feel like Superman. You're flying. Ideas come at the speed of light. You go 72 hours straight without so much as a coffee break. You don't need sleep; you don't need nourishment. If it's sex you're after, you go all night.... Then you crash. It's like falling down a well or parachuting without a parachute. You go running back. You're looking for the German mosquito, the insect with the magic pinprick. He stings you, and all at once you're soaring again.[1]

Capote described Jacobson as a "powerful theatrical figure," but stopped going to him after a series of treatments. What he needed was a break. He would go on a journey. His whole soul was bent on fame. He moved to Paris. He told others he wanted to get away because he had collapsed and had to be hospitalized after a period of steady amphetamine use by Jacobson. The typical withdrawal reaction is a sudden and extreme depression and physical lethargy. Capote said the injections were supposed to be special vitamins but that because of the way he had felt, he was sure they were loaded with "speed."[2]

He finally returned from Paris, but many avoided him. He was again lonely and stupidly used drugs despite his earlier hospitalization. Stupidity is the sin that is never forgiven and always punished. Truman Capote died in the Bel Air home of Joanne Carson (ex-wife of NBC's *Tonight Show* host, Johnny Carson) from drug intoxication in addition to liver disease and phlebitis.

Notes

1. C. David Heymann, *A Woman Named Jackie*. New York: Carol Communications, 1989, page 301.
2. https://www.nytimes.com/1972/12/04/archives/amphetamines-used-by-a-physician-to-lift-moods-of-famous-patients.html) *The New York Times*, Dec. 4, 1972. by Boyce Rensberger.

Van Cliburn

Harry Lavan "Van" Cliburn, Jr. (1934-2013) was an American pianist born in Louisiana to an oil executive and piano teacher. His mother discovered him playing at the age of three mimicking one of her students. She arranged for him to start taking lessons with the best teachers they could afford. His hands grew large, and he was easily able to play octaves and more with each hand. They moved to Texas where oil was plentiful for his father's career, and Van began to play and win local Texas piano competitions.

His parents believed he was going to be a star, so his mother trained him to serve dinner to them. She thought that if he grew up as one who serves others, he would not be too full of himself. He remained a humble man who served classical music to others winning numerous competitions. He began to treat those he met as if they were the most important people in the world.

She also taught her son to sing the music he was going to play. It became a song in his head that came out through his mouth and his fingertips onto the piano keys. He often closed his eyes as he played, thinking all the while of the effect he wanted to establish.

He entered the Juilliard School of Musical in New York City when he was seventeen, where he was trained him in the tradition of the great Russian romantic musicians. He made his debut at Carnegie Hall at age twenty. By this time, the lanky Texan had reached his full height of six feet four inches tall, with a mop of wavy hair.

He was pushed on every side to great achievement. He never knew the sweet idleness of youth. Bearing the burden of his genius, he performed to great applause, hampered only by fear of failure in front of an audience—stagefright.

During the Cold War, the Russians launched Sputnik in October 1957, demonstrating their lead in the technological era. Suddenly, it looked to the world as if Russia was far ahead of America in the field of electronics and jet-propelled aircraft. Russia decided to show the world that their power extended even to culture, so they created the International Tchaikovsky Piano Competition in 1958. It was expected to demonstrate Russian cultural superiority to the world.

Cliburn's teacher at the Julliard School of Music encouraged young Cliburn to compete. He was extremely modest, shy, and anxious. Each competition was anxiety-provoking for him. His piano was the main way he could touch people, so he worked extremely hard to prepare himself for this competition. By this time, he had established a homosexual relationship and worried that this would become known.

At the age of twenty-three, Van Cliburn flew to Moscow where he played Tchaikovsky's *Piano Concerto No. 1* and *Rachmaninoff's Piano Concerto No. 3* on April 13, 1958, earning him a standing ovation. He made some brief comments in Russian, resumed his seat at the piano, and began to play his own arrangement of the beloved *Moscow Nights*, which further endeared him to the Russian audience. The Russians loved him. The surprised judges felt they must ask Soviet leader Nikita Khrushchev in the audience about whether they should award the prize to an American.

Khrushchev asked, "Is he the best? Then, give it to him." Cliburn became world-famous at that moment. The press gave him the nickname "America's Sputnik." He came back to the United States where a New York City ticker tape parade was held, and the tall Texan became the only musician ever honored by such a parade.

Everyone wanted him to appear. The Steve Allen *Tonight Show* asked him to appear. He became frozen with anxiety backstage. Dr. Max Jacobson was summoned to reduce his anxiety and shaky hands with an injection of "liquid vitamins" and he was able to come out, interview, and play for the audience. This began a long tradition of delaying his appearances before audiences for up to an hour or more. He silently questioned whether applause was a kind of sympathy, as if the audience shared a secret of wanting to be better than they were. But they were his enemies, because they would be judging his every note.

Nigel Cliff wrote *Moscow Nights* and Stuart Isacoff wrote *When the World Stopped To Listen: Van Cliburn's Cold War Triumph, and Its Aftermath,* published by Knopf in 2017. Isacoff recounted the 1958 victory and Cliburn's "blow-up" during his rehearsal to appear on the Steve Allen Show in May 1958. The author also described the relief that Dr. Max Jacobson provided with an injection.

When Van returned to Texas, he wound up playing for royalty, heads of state, and every president from Harry Truman down to Barack Obama. But he was changing, gradually coming to hate the strain of such important appearances. Not that he was doing bad work, but he got no joy in it. As time passed, he made only rare appearances and lived a quiet homosexual life. In public, he put on a courtly attitude to hide his bitter struggles with his loneliness.

Toward the end, his partner Thomas Smith cared for him when he became ill with bone cancer until his death. He had performed at Texas Christian University several times and that institution developed the Van Cliburn piano competition that continues to this day. Stuart Cheney, the Division Chair of Musicology at TCU described the continued popularity of those Van Cliburn competitions.

Rosemary Clooney

Rosemary Clooney (1928-2002) was an American singer and actress, born to Irish Catholics in Kentucky. Rosemary and sister Betty became entertainers and her brother, Nick, became a newsman and TV broadcaster. In 1945, the Clooney sisters were hired by a radio station as singers. Rosemary cut several records for songs and became famous singing "Come On-a My House" in 1951. She appeared on television and radio shows.

In 1953, she married movie actor Jose Ferrer born in San Juan, Puerto Rico, whose first two wives were actress Uta Hagen and singer Phyllis Hill. Rosemary starred in the 1954 movie *White Christmas* with Bing Crosby, Danny Kaye, and Vera-Ellen. In 1956, she had a 30-minute musical variety show on television called *The Rosemary Clooney Show*. She and Crosby became friends and sang together frequently. She starred on television shows and occasionally appeared with her nephew, actor George Clooney.

Here are some lines from *White Christmas:*
"Why, all of a sudden, are people so concerned about my eating habits? Why don't people just leave me alone?"

Singing "I Wish I Was Back in the Army," she sang: "The soldiers and the WACS/The WACs who dressed in slacks/Dancing check-to-cheek and pants-to-pants."

Rosemary and Jose had five children, and one of them was Gabriel who married Debby Boone, daughter of Pat and Shirley Boone. Debby followed in her father's footsteps as a singer and became famous with her 1977 song, *You Light Up My Life*.

By the early 1960s, Rosemary had a demanding career, five children at home, and an unfaithful husband.

Stress built up and she began taking prescription drugs, barbiturates, and alcohol. She and Jose both had injections from Dr. Max Jacobson and recommended him to others. She became addicted. With unpredictable behavior, Rosemary's voice declined, and her career was cut short.

She divorced Ferrer in 1961, but they remarried in 1964 until 1967. After their first divorce, Jose was willing to try again. She had to make a guess about whether anything would be better. A guess is either right or wrong. If it is right, we call it intuition. If it is wrong, we try to never mention it again. Their drug use and drinking continued. Clooney's nephew George has stated his reluctance to take painkillers because of the family history of addiction.

In 1968, Rosemary suffered a nervous breakdown. She had been working hard in Robert Kennedy's campaign for the presidency and was only a few feet away when he was killed at the Ambassador Hotel. At this point, Clooney was aware that she needed help and agreed to receive treatment, which did help her get into a more stable place mentally and emotionally.

According to the *Washington Post*, "Rosemary Clooney Suffered a Nervous Breakdown" by Michael Ochs, she said, "Nobody could approach me. I was like a hand grenade with the pin pulled. Nobody could tell whether it was a dud or the real thing, because one minute I could be completely sweet and kind, the next, a raving monster."

Upon admission to a hospital psychiatric unit, she was diagnosed with addiction and bipolar disorder. In one of her autobiographies, she recalled this experience saying: "My brink of despair was rushing up to meet me like the end of a runway for a plane lumbering in vain to get off the ground." She was also disturbed by her considerable weight gain.

She made a comeback in 1977, when Bing Crosby asked her to appear with him in a show marking his 50th anniversary in show business. She continued recording until her death in 2002 from lung cancer due to smoking.

She married Dante DiPaolo in 1997, her long-time friend and dance partner, and lived for some years in Beverly Hills, California, in a home formerly owned by George and Ira Gershwin. That house has since been demolished.[1,2]

Notes

1. https://www.grunge.com/298610/the-tragic-true-story-of-rosemary-clooney/
2. See her two autobiographies: *This for Remembrance: The Autobiography of Rosemary Clooney, an Irish-American Singer* published in 1977 with a preface by Bing Crosby, and *Girl Singer: An Autobiography* published in 2001.

Robert Cummings

Robert (Bob) Cummings (1910-1990) was an American film and TV actor who was born to a surgeon and his wife, a minister of the Science of the Mind. Thus, from childhood, he heard of medical problems that could be cut out by a surgeon and strange ways to consider the mind.

Many came to hear his mother orate about her religion which was like Christian Scientists who believed physical health could be obtained through prayer rather than scientific doctors. Thus, many souls were not stirred by such orators.

While attending high school, Bob learned to fly in 1927, the year of his first solo flight. He occasionally gave Joplin, Missouri, residents a ride in his airplane for $5 per person.[1]

After graduating high school, he began studying at Drury College in Missouri and transferred to Carnegie Institute of Technology in Pittsburgh where he studied aeronautical engineering until his father lost funds in the 1929 stock market crash. He became interested in acting and trained at the American Academy of Dramatic Arts in New York City where he learned the basics.

He married Emma Mayers in 1931 in a wedding ceremony conducted by his mother, but they divorced in 1933.

Bob began looking for roles as an actor and found that English accents and actors were in demand. He moved to England where he invented a stage name: Blade Stanhope Conway. He had pictures taken of himself and sent them to New York pretending to be an Englishman. Finally, he landed a role in the Laurel and Hardy 1933 comedy *Songs of the Desert*. Then he took another stage name, Bryce Hutchens, and appeared in *Ziegfeld Follies of 1934*.

Robert wanted to be somebody. He then heard that Texas movie producer King Vidor, longest movie director ever (1913-1980) was looking for Texans for his 1935 movie *So Red the Rose* starring Margaret Sullivan and Randolph Scott. Cummings appeared in that movie under his real name, Robert Cummings. Vidor, born in Galveston, Texas, of Hungarian parentage, directed the film and went on to make many big hits.[2]

He married Vivi Janiss in 1935 until 1943 and served as a flight instructor after joining the United States Army Air Forces. He was in many movies during that era.[3] Cummings also starred in two Alfred Hitchcock movies, first in 1942 *Saboteur* and then later in 1954 *Dial M for Murder.* Here are some of his lines from the latter movie with Ray Milland and Grace Kelly:

> Milland: "How do you go about writing a detective story?"
> Cummings: "Well, you forget detection and concentrate on crime. Crime's the thing. And then you imagine you're going to steal something or murder somebody."
> Kelly: "Let me get you another drink, Mark, before Tony comes. I ought to explain something."
> Cummings: "Yes, I've been waiting for that."
> Kelly: "I haven't told him anything about us."

In 1945, Cummings appeared in *You Came Along* with a screenplay by Ayn Rand. By then, Rand had been using amphetamines for three years and would use them for some thirty years before her death. Perhaps the actor and author talked about the value they placed on the energizing substance.[4] She used an amphetamine when she needed to complete a movie of her book *The Fountainhead* in record time and became addicted.[5]

Cummings married Mary Elliott in 1945, and that marriage would last until 1970. Some of Bob's movies were flops but he appeared in the film noir 1948 *Sleep, My Love*, and a romantic comedy with Hedy Lamarr in the 1948 *Let's Live a Little*. Around 1950, Cummings began working in television. His appearances went so well that he starred in his first regular television series called *My Hero* which ran for 33 episodes from 1952-1953.

In 1954, Cummings joined the Civil Air Patrol, where citizens and pilots helped support the U.S. war effort. He participated in search and rescue missions, using his own aircraft, Spinach I and later a Spinach II. He also formed his own movie production company in 1954, where his wife was appointed president of Laurel Productions, named after their daughter Laurel.

Despite having been an extremely healthy vitamin consumer, Bob felt a loss of pep. His friends, Rosemary Clooney and Jose Ferrer, recommended Dr. Max Jacobson who gave vitamin shots that made them feel full of pep. He began a routine of using Jacobson's injections and would go on to use Jacobson's son for his supplies later. Throughout his life, Cummings used astrology and unusual methods to make decisions about what to do, which must have come from his mother's work as a psychic or minister of the mind. Was he led astray by using what sounded like scientific information, but was not?

In 1955, he began *The Bob Cummings Show* which aired on television through 1959 with co-stars Rosemary DeCamp, Dwayne Hickman, and Ann Davis. He won an Emmy for his show in 1956 and made many other television shows. In 1959, he announced that he would take a year off and consider further projects. He starred in some more movies and began another sitcom called *My Living Doll*, co-starring Julie Newmar as a robot, but after 21 episodes, asked to be written out of the show or was fired. Julie had watched him inject himself in his ankles. Bob took Dwayne to Dr. Jacobson's office and asked him to get a shot, but Hickman declined.[6]

He continued to be on television, made more movies and wrote *Stay Young and Vital* published in 1960. That book offered to build vitality, enthusiasm, and youthfulness at any age.

Gradually, he was losing his way as he became more addicted to the amphetamines with the Jacobson injections. His friends and cast members noted changes in his behavior. His dear friend Art Linkletter, a Canadian born radio and television personality, had a daughter who committed suicide due to drugs and became an anti-drug advocate. Linkletter's shows and his book "Kids Say the Darnedest Things" were best-sellers. Art tried to reason with Cummings about his drug addiction, but it was useless.[7]

Bob's wife Mary Elliott divorced him in 1970 claiming that he cheated on her with his former secretary and that he had wild mood swings due to his methamphetamine use. He did marry that secretary, Regina Fong, the following year on a date agreed upon by three astrologers. Their marriage lasted until 1987.[8]

When Dr. Max Jacobson was forced out of business in 1970, Cummings developed his own line of vitamins based in the Bahamas.[9] Articles appeared in the paper with accusations and convictions of Jacobson. Bob may have thought he had fallen into the clutches of a criminal, but he became a criminal himself.

In 1952, Cummings was sued by the writer of *My Hero* who had been fired. In 1952, Cummings was served with papers concerning a lawsuit by LA County Deputy Sheriff William Conroy; Cummings assaulted Conroy and was then sued by the sheriff for damages. Conroy stated that when he tried to serve Cummings with a subpoena, the actor gunned the motor of his car and dragged him along the pavement. Cummings explained that he didn't know Conroy was a deputy. In 1972 he was charged with fraud for operating a pyramid scheme involving his company, Bob Cummings Inc, which sold vitamins and food supplements. In 1975 he was arrested for being in possession of a blue box used to defraud the telephone company. Details can be found under his name in Wikipedia.

He was in some TV movies, and he traveled about in an Airstream travel trailer for dinner theater productions. He had some cameo roles and hosted the 1986 Walt Disney World on *The Wonderful World of Disney*. In 1987, He made this statement:

> I wouldn't mind living until I'm 110. I still swim, do calisthenics, and keep fit... People laugh about my using so many vitamins... I'm retired, I live on a pension... and if I have a problem I get expert counsel, then ask the opinion of a good psychic."[10]

When that marriage with Elliott ended because of his drug use, he had several relationships that fizzled until he was very ill. He then married Martha Burzynski in 1989.

He died a few months later at the Motion Picture and Television Hospital in Woodland Hills, California. His death resulted from kidney failure and complications of pneumonia. He also suffered from Parkinson's Disease and was living in a home for indigent older actors in Hollywood before admission to the hospital. He had seven children from his five marriages.[11]

Notes

1. http://walkoffame.com and http://nla.gov.au/nia.news-article222144042)
2. *A Tree Is a Tree* by King Vidor, 1954, Longmans, Green and Co. Ltd., England, page 214.
3. http://airforce.togetherweserved.com/usaf/servlet/tws.WebApp?cmd=ShadowBoxProfile&type=Person&ID=113400
4. "Ayn Rand: Speed Addict? Theweek.com/articles/493764/ayn-rand-speed-addict
5. https://www.ibtimes.com/mad-men-meets-dr-feelgood-sterling-cooper-draper-pryce-drugs-1271003
6. Newmarnews.blogspot.com/2020/08/don't-love-that-bob.html
7. *R.I.P. Art Linkletter, Who Got Kids to Say the Darnedest Things* by Sean O'Neal, 2010.
8. "Robert Cummings Divorced" *The New York Times*. January 16, 1970, p. 33, ProQuest 118877797 https://search.proquest.com/docview/118877797
9. "Actor Cummings, Cosmetics Magnate Charged with Fraud" *Los Angeles Times*, by Alexander Auerbach, September 26, 1972, page 3.
10. *The Dr. Feelgood Casebook: Max Jacobson: Einstein or Frankenstein* by William J. Birnes and Richard A. Lertzman, 2016, Brilliance Audio

11. Flint, Peter B. December 4, 1990. "Robert Cummings is dead at 82; Debonair actor in TV and films." https:www.nytimes.com/1990/12/04/obituaries/robert-cummings-is-dead-at-82-debonair-actor-in-tv-and-films.html

Cecile B. DeMille

Cecile B. DeMille (1881-1959) made about seventy movies, both silent and sound films. His productions were distinguished by the epic scale and his showmanship. His father was an English teacher at Columbia College and his mother worked as a literary agent and scriptwriter. His parents were members of a music and literary society in New York. He watched his father and famed impresario and director David Belasco rehearse their Broadway plays including the Puccini story of *Madame Butterfly*. Belasco became famous when he produced the first *Madame Butterfly* production for the stage.

DeMille also recalled a lunch with his father and actor Edwin Booth, brother of actor John Wilkes Booth who killed President Lincoln. With such distinguished family stories, he "thought big" from the beginning of his life.

DeMIlle was the first director to make movies in Hollywood, after trying to film *Squaw Man* in Arizona. Near the Grand Canyon, mountains were so foreboding that he found no plains for his scenes, so he moved his 1914 cast to what is now called Hollywood. He made that movie three times and it was highly successful.

DeMille's first two *Squaw Man* movies were silent, and his third was made in Castle Hot Springs near Phoenix, Arizona, at the resort where John Kennedy stayed for his health in 1945. DeMille brought his cast including Warner Baxter, Lupe Velez, and Charles Bickford to that resort for filming. DeMille told Philip K. Scheur of the *Los Angeles Times* on September 14, 1930:

> My next picture is hokum—beautiful hokum. It is *The Squaw Man*. An American *Madame Butterfly*.

I have made it twice before. But now, with words it will be twice as poignant.

He simply could not forget those early memories from his father's time when *Madame Butterfly* was a big hit on stage. People called him "old-fashioned", but they went to his movies. DeMille narrated his films, appeared in their trailers, carried a megaphone, riding crop, and wore jodhpurs. He played himself in movies such as Billy Wilder's 1950 *Sunset Boulevard* where actress Gloria Swanson spoke to DeMille saying, "All right, I'm ready for my close up, Mr. DeMIlle."[1]

DeMille filmed movies from the *Bible* four times: 1923 and 1956 *The Ten Commandments*, 1927 *The King of Kings*, and 1949 *Samson and Delilah*. In fact, his second *The Ten Commandments* was shown annually for thirty years on ABC TV.

DeMille helped blacklisted artists return to work. Edward G. Robinson wrote, "Cecil B. DeMille returned me to films. Cecil B. DeMille restored my self-respect." Academy Award winning composer Elmer Bernstein scored the 1956 version of *The Ten Commandments* said that he owed DeMille "everything."[2] He helped actors get big breaks such as Charlton Heston whom he cast in 1952 *The Greatest Show on Earth*. He was in touch with what movie audiences wanted in his epic films.

DeMille not only made movies but hosted the Lux Radio Theater from 1935 to 1954. This was one of the most popular radio shows in history, with some forty million listeners every Monday night.

He suffered an emergency prostatectomy in 1939 and suffered from sexual dysfunction for the rest of his life, ending his infidelities during marriage. His health and age rendered him unable to serve in WWII, but he was a neighborhood air-raid warden. In the 1950s, he was recruited by Allen Dulles to serve on the board of the anti-communist National Committee for a Free Europe that oversaw Radio Free Europe service. His adopted daughter, Katherine, became an actress and married actor Anthony Quinn in 1936.

DeMille's final film was *The Ten Commandments* and the Exodus scene was filmed on-site in Egypt, as well other scenes filmed in Paris and Hollywood. The cast included people like Charlton Heston, Yul Brynner, Edward G. Robinson, Yvonne De Carlo, John Derek, Sir Cedric Hardwick, Nina Foch, Vincent Price, and John Carradine and Dr. Jacobson oversaw their medical needs and kept people working with his amphetamine injections. DeMille thought Jacobson's injections made people peppy so they worked longer, thus he brought Max to Egypt with the cast.

DeMille had heart problems and suffered a heart attack while ascending a ladder on November 7, 1954. The 73-year-old director wanted to check a high camera, so he stayed atop a scaffold. His assistant producer actor Henry Wilcoxon climbed up the ladder to hold him so he would not fall. He told DeMille that he must come down and go to the hospital. DeMille slapped Wilcoxon away saying, "Who the hell do you think you are? No one tells me what to do!"[3]

Wilcoxon and Katherine DeMille Quinn took over as directors. Cecil got better and continued to direct while reducing his physical stress. DeMille had a vision about this movie, and only he could make it happen.

In Egypt, De Mille was like an archaeologist. When something comes up out of the ground in an excavation, everything is cleared away very carefully around it. Finally, your object is there with no extraneous matter confusing it. That is what he was seeking to do, present clear evidence that God exists, demonstrate stones with laws commanded by God, and part the Red Sea in a miracle which only God could perform. He played God.

DeMille skillfully directed large crowds, thousands of extras, train wrecks, and the parting of the Red Sea in *The Ten Commandments*. That scene was created by releasing 360,000 gallons of water into a huge water tank split by a U-shaped trough, overlaying it with a film of a giant waterfall that was built on the studio back lot, and played the clip backwards. There was no one to be compared to him. His movies were major spectacles because he thought "Bigger is better!"

Cecil B. DeMille later travelled to Italy with his daughter and Dr. Max Jacobson. They met with Pope Pius XII on October 9, 1957, at his summer residence, and there is a famous photograph of the four of them standing together. He was a very religious man.

DeMille had almost finished his autobiography when he died, and it was published in November 1959. He left his huge estate to daughter Cecilia because his wife had Alzheimer's dementia and she soon died.[4]

Notes

1. https://www.cecilbdemill.com/legacy/
2. https://www.cecilbdemille.com/legacy/
3. autocratonasofa.com/2020/12/27/the-ten-commandments-cecil-b-de-mille-1956-part-8/
4. *Autobiography of Cecile B. DeMille* published by Prentice Hall, New York; New York: Prentice Hall, 1959.

Marlene Dietrich

Marie Magdalene "Marlene" Dietrich (1901-1992) was born in Berlin, Germany, and died in Paris, France. Her mother was from an affluent family who owned a jewelry and clock-making firm, and her father was a police lieutenant and she had one sister. She studied violin but a wrist injury ended her thoughts of becoming a concert violinist. Young Marlene became a chorus girl and played small roles in theaters and movies. Her name was pronounced Marlena so her nickname when young was Lena. Dietrich was pronounced, Deetrish.

She was in the 1923 movie *The Little Napoleon* where she met her future husband Rudolf Sieber, an assistant movie director. They had one daughter, Maria Riva, born in 1924. Dietrich worked in more movies until her big breakthrough in 1930 with *The Blue Angel* starring Emil Jannings. Her husband introduced her to director Josef von Sternberg, and he included Dietrich's signature song "Falling in Love Again." He went on to direct her as a glamorous femme fatale, which led to her discovery in American films.

Marlene lived with her husband for only five years, but they never divorced. She was so grateful to him for her career that she maintained him on his chicken ranch in California until his death in 1976.

In 1930, she starred with Gary Cooper in *Morocco* as a cabaret singer. She performed a song dressed like a man and kissed a woman, earning her only Academy Award nomination. She was bisexual and had relations with men and women throughout her life. Marlene starred in the 1932 *Blonde Venus* with Cary Grant and was in the extravagant 1934 movie *The Scarlet Empress*. Director von Sternberg used light and shadow to bring out her beauty and talent.

Marlene starred in the color film of 1936 entitled *The Garden of Allah*, produced by David O. Selznick. In 1937, Dietrich she was asked by Nazi Party officials to return to Germany as a foremost film star but refused their offers and applied for American citizenship that year. She starred in the 1939 western *Destry Rides Again* opposite James Stewart. Her song "See What the Boys in the Back Room Will Have" became a hit which she recorded.

She went on to be in the 1940 *Seven Sinners* and 1942 movie *The Spoilers* with John Wayne. Here are some quotes from *Seven Sinners*:

Wayne: "Imagine finding you here."

Dietrich: "I'm the type of girl you're liable to find anywhere."
Officer: "There've been a half-dozen complaints since you came to that café."
Dietrich: "A half dozen? Why not fifty? I'm surprised."

Marlene and John Wayne had a three-year affair. Like any lover, he desired to please. So, they had an epic rendezvous on the staircase of the Excelsior Hotel in Rome one evening. Yes, as he said, "I took her on the staircase." Wayne called it the best sexual experience of his life. She had other brief sexual encounters with Ambassador Joseph Kennedy, President John Kennedy, and too many others to name.

By 1942, Marlene had created a fund with director Billy Wilder and other exiles to help Jews and dissidents escape from Germany. In 1941, she became one of the first public figures to help sell war bonds, toured to entertain US troops, and sold more war bonds than any other star. She performed in Algeria, Italy, the United Kingdom, France, and the Netherlands.

She entered Germany with Generals James M. Gavin and George S. Patton. In 1944, the OSS (Office of Strategic Services) initiated musical propaganda broadcasts to demoralize enemy soldiers and she sang songs in German such as "Lili Marleen," a favorite of soldiers on both sides in WWI. Major General William J. Donovan, head of the OSS, wrote her saying "I am personally deeply grateful for your generosity in making these recordings for us."[1] At last, she was a woman of significance.

Dietrich received the Medal of Freedom in 1947 for her "extraordinary record entertaining troops overseas during the war and was also awarded by the Franch government for her wartime work.

Marlene preserved her glamorous image for so many years that her health began to suffer. She was operated on for cervical cancer in 1965 and depended upon painkillers and alcohol to continue her work. She began to use the services of Max Jacobson to enliven her performances. The German actress disliked his messy office and used a broom to clean it up.

As time passed, she injured her leg and skin grafts were required to allow the wound to heal. She broke her right leg in 1974. The following year, when she fell on stage in Australia, she broke a thigh bone. Her husband on the chicken farm died of cancer the following year. Marlene's final appearance was a brief scene in the 1979 movie *Just a Gigolo* where she sang the title song.

She moved to a Paris apartment where she was bedridden for the last thirteen years of her life, seeing mainly family and employees. She was quite a letter writer, and her autobiography *Take Just My Life*, was published in 1979. She agreed to participate in a documentary about her life (1984 *Marlene*) but did not want to be filmed, so actor/director Maximilian Schell interviewed her and recorded her voice. It won an Academy Award nomination for the Best Documentary in 1985.

She remained in contact with world leaders by telephone such as Ronald Reagan, Mikhail Gorbachev, and Margaret Thatcher, running up huge telephone bills. Such are the diversions of important people. They ring up anybody and everybody. She spoke about the fall of the Berlin Wall in 1989 and spoke with former French president Mitterrand regarding his promise to her that Berlin would be the capital city of a united Germany.

She died of kidney failure in Paris age the age of ninety on May 6, 1992. Her funeral was attended by international mourners and her coffin was adorned with flowers from French President Francois Mitterand.

Note

1. *Sisterhood of Spies: The Women of the OSS* by Elizabeth P. McIntosh, 1998, London: Dell Publishers, p. 59.
   See also: https://www.bookforum.com/print/1403/-855 *Dietrich Icon*, ed. Elisabeth Bronfen, Joseph Garncarz, Patrice Petro, Eric Rentschler, Duke University Press, 2007.

Eddie Fisher

Edwin Jack Fisher was born (1928-2010) in Philadelphia to a Jewish grocer and his wife from the Russian Empire whose name was originally Tisch. He began singing early at synagogue and school and dropped out of high school to follow a singing career. He won amateur contests and performed on the Arthur Godfrey Talent Scouts radio show. By 1946, he was crooning in bands and was heard in 1949 by Eddie Cantor in the Catskills Resort Hotel where Fisher began to record songs.

He was drafted into the Army in 1951, served a year in Korea, and became the official soloist for the U.S. Army Band. Eddie was popular among teenagers, having 17 songs in the Top Ten between 1950 and 1956. He married Debbie Reynolds in 1955, and they appeared in the movie *Bundle of Joy*. They were married for four years and had Carrie and Todd Fisher.

Fisher starred in 1960 *Butterfield 8*, for which Elizabeth Taylor won an Academy Award for Best Actress. Here is some dialogue from two scenes in that movie:

> Taylor: I always said I'd try anything once.
> Fisher: Ever try common sense?
> Taylor: Only in desperation.
> Fisher: What does your analyst say about all this?
> Taylor: Oh, I only tell Dr. Tredman what I think he ought to hear.
> Fish: Oh, that's very intelligent.
> Taylor: If I were intelligent, I wouldn't need a psychiatrist.

He was best friends with movie producer Mike Todd who was married to Elizabeth Taylor, and he consoled the widow after Todd died in a plane crash. That grew into more of a relationship, and he left Debbie to marry Elizabeth. This caused much controversy, and his TV Eddie Fisher Show was canceled in 1959. His marriage to Taylor lasted from 1959 to 1964, when she began an affair with Richard Burton while filming *Cleopatra*.

Fisher married singer Connie Stevens from 1967 to 1969. Their short-lived marriage brought two daughters, Joely and Tricia. He then married beauty queen Terry Richard for a few months and that ended with his extreme drug abuse and gambling debts.

Fisher's daughter, Joely wrote *Growing Up Fisher: Musings, Memories and Misadventures,* which described her youth with Eddie Fisher and Connie Stevens. She saw her father putting drugs into his arm and described her mother having an affair with singer Elvis Presley. Carrie Fisher wrote about her life while suffering from and being treated for a manic-depressive disorder. At the end of Carrie's life, her mother Debbie Reynolds also died within the same week after their reunion of sorts.

Fisher wrote two autobiographies: *My Life, My Loves* and *Been There Done That*. The latter book described his life including his relationship with Max Jacobson. He said that he and President John Kennedy shared a more sinister bond as they were both patients of Dr. Max Jacobson.[1]

He stated that he began to use Jacobson's serum at age 25 when he was having trouble with his voice prior to a performance. That first shot of methamphetamine hooked Fisher for 37 years, or so he said. He wrote of Jacobson:

> He was a very big figure in my life... I think he thought he was helping people, but I think he got

terribly, terribly lost in the middle of it all... I think the medication went to his brain because he used 100 times more than he used on us guinea pigs. He would give himself these injections and he would fall asleep in the middle of injecting us. But I didn't know it at the time. I figured he was a doctor, and he was so famous and what he did for me—in my mind, I thought I was more brilliant than I was. I didn't know that I was an idiot. And he made me sing better, I thought. But I discovered years later when I was no longer on methamphetamine that I sang better without it.

Fisher had thought of returning home, returning to reason, self-mastery, an ordered existence. He tried to make a comeback in the 1980s but failed as he suffered from various problems such as knee, back, hearing, and eyesight. In this middle-aged man's mind, these physical defects seemed a shameful thing.

Fisher's last marriage was to Chinese businesswoman Betty Lin from 1993 until her death in 2001. In that marriage, he got off drugs. Apparently, Fisher responded to love in a way that he never would have to knowledge or psychology. His "teacher" cared about him, and he blossomed. Betty was a wealthy Asian family-oriented woman who encouraged him to reunite with his children. After her death, he interacted more with his children who finally had to care for him as he aged.

Note

1. www.ccn.com/books/news/9910/04/eddie.fisher/

John and Jacqueline Kennedy

John Fitzgerald Kennedy (1917-1963) was born to politician and businessman, Joseph Kennedy Sr. and his wife Rose. His paternal grandfather had served as a Massachusetts state legislator and his maternal grandfather was a U.S. Congressman and Mayor of Boston. His family was of Irish heritage, and he had eight siblings.

John's health problems ruled his life. At age two, he contracted scarlet fever on the day his mother gave birth to his sister, Kathleen. Fearing he might transmit the fever to his sibling, he was rushed to Boston City Hospital. He became so sick that a priest was called in to deliver last rights. But he pulled through and received treatment for six weeks, then spent six weeks in isolation until he could return home.[1]

John became a sickly youth with a weakened immune system that made him slow to recover from childhood and other illnesses. Unlike his brothers who were taught by their father to compete physically and mentally, he was seen as less able to do so. He was a challenge for his parents, teachers, and doctors. His life was so precarious from early childhood and required so many treatments of various kinds that he became a "devil-may-care" reckless youth.

At age 14 he attended Choate School, a prestigious boarding school in Connecticut. His IQ was 119 when he was tested before entrance, according to biographer Robert Dallek's *An Unfinished Life: John F. Kennedy, 1917-1963*, published in 2004. Assassin Lee Harvey Oswald was tested at age 13 in a psychiatric institution and found to have an IQ of 118, thus both John and Lee had a bright average intelligence.

At Choate, he and school chum Lem Billings pulled tricks and were nearly expelled. The Kennedy sons knew that their father had many affairs outside of marriage to well-known women who sometimes visited their house. Those affairs included actresses Gloria Swanson, Marlene Dietrich, and a secretary. Thus, his sons followed him in such pursuits and Kennedy began having sexual adventures quite early.

At age 19, his father sent John and older brother Joe to the Jay Six dude ranch in Benson, Arizona, for a summer to toughen up frail John. By this time, he was often called Jack. The boys built an office for the boss and tended horses. Jack slipped across the nearby border several times with a male friend to have unprotected sex with Mexican prostitutes. He required treatment for gonorrhea then and later in his life. He described that in letters to chum Lem Billings which can be found in *JFK: Reckless Youth* by Nigel Hamilton, published in 1992 by Random House. There is a letter he wrote Lem in May 1936 which he entitled "Travels in a Mexican Whore-house with Your Roomie" and he signed himself "your gonnereick roomie."

When Jack was twenty-one, his father took the family on vacation at Hotel du Cap near Cannes, France, in August 1938. Joseph had served six months as Ambassador in England. He had a habit of inviting his paramours to his home and his wife did nothing about that. So, John Kennedy saw his father going into Marlene Dietrich's cabana. Her husband was aware that she was bisexual and didn't worry too much about her disappearance from time to time. When John became president, he invited Marlene to the White House when she was doing her one-woman show nearby. They had a quickie, and she was ready to go back to the theater when he asked if she had sex with his father. She merely said, "He tried." Obviously, the Kennedy boys followed their father's example when it came to women.[2]

John graduated from Harvard University in 1940. He wrote a college thesis called in 1940 called *Why England Slept*. His father disagreed with his son's ideas but wanted fame for the lad so had his friends help do a foreword and rewrite it so that it could be published in 1940.

John joined the U.S. Naval Reserve the following year. While serving as an ensign, he met Danish journalist Inga Arvad, who was living with his sister Kathleen, called Kick, in Washington, D.C.

Arvad was a beautiful young journalist who had married a man in 1931. After their divorce, she married a Hungarian film director in 1936 and starred in three movies. She was invited by Adolf Hitler to the summer Olympics in 1936 where she interviewed him. She was thought to be a potential spy by the FBI when she came to America as a journalist.[3]

When Kathleen introduced them, Jack and Inga were immediately attracted to each other and began dating. By then, the FBI was checking Inga wondering if she was a Nazi spy. They spoke with John's superior officer since he was working in the Naval Reserves intelligence office looking over documents. They decided to transfer him to Charleston, South Carolina, just in case she was a spy.

FBI agents were tapping her phone and learned that she was making trips to Charleston so they could be together. They stayed at a particular hotel and agents put listening devices under their bed at J. Edgar Hoover's insistence. While no important intelligence information was passed, some comments were made. Kennedy's superior officer was advised, and John was transferred to a seagoing unit since they were still unsure whether Arvad was a spy.[4]

Inga and John exchanged letters which can be seen at https://www.jfklibrary.org/asset-viewer/archives/JFKPP/004/JFKPP-004-052. Those letters show that she was very much aware of his bad back and frequent pain, which may have interfered with his bodily positions during intercourse. Kennedy's Catholic father told him to stop the affair, as she was a divorcee. Jack told her about that just before his transfer to the Pacific Theater.

During WWII, he commanded a PT boat in the Pacific theater, survived its sinking, and although wounded, rescued fellow sailors, earning him the Navy and Marine Corps medal. When Kennedy returned to the United States, Arvad helped to make him a hero by her story of January 13, 1944, in *The Pittsburgh Press*. Here is the beginning of that article:

"Lt. Kennedy Saves His Men as Japs Cut PT Boat in Half. All but two returned after destroyer rams them" by Inga Arvad.

This is a story of the 13 American men on PT boat 109 who got closer than any others to a Japanese destroyer and of the 11 who lived to tell about it. It is about the skipper hero, 26-year-old Lt. John F. Kennedy, son of Joseph Kennedy, former U.S. ambassador to Great Britain, now home on leave, who thought he saved three lives, and swam for long hours in shark-infested waters to rescue his men, today says: 'None of that hero stuff about me. The real heroes are not the men who return, but those who stay out there like plenty of them do, two of my men included.[5]

There was no doubt that his courage in battle saved lives. He was wounded but he served his men well.

Jack and Arvad continued to correspond lovingly as she signed her name Binga, so Kennedy referred to her as Inga Binga. Arvad went on with her life and was hired by David O. Selznick to promote 1945 *Duel in the Sun* by traveling across the country. She worked for MGM and met wealthy cowboy actor Tim McCoy whom she married in 1946 until her death in 1973 near Nogales, Arizona. Author Seymour Hersh wrote about her affair with Kennedy in his 1997 *The Dark Side of Camelot*.

Following the death of John's brother Joseph in August 1944 in a naval airplane explosion, old Joe wanted John to prepare for the presidency. Being quite sick after his PT boat service, his father sent him to Castle Hot Springs, Arizona, for rest and recuperation beginning in January 1945. Treated with the curative waters in that site, proper food with meat sent by his father, he gradually healed. The treatment center, which is now a high-class dude ranch near Lake Pleasant in the Phoenix area, attracts a well-heeled clientele.

In April 1945, John left treatment and was given an assignment by William Randoph Hearst thanks to Joseph Kennedy's intervention. Hearst asked John to write on topics such as the founding of the United Nations. Kennedy's writing was poor and needed spelling and grammatical corrections, but it gave him exposure. Later, aide Ted Sorenson wrote his speeches and papers with great aplomb. For example, "Ask not what your country can do for you, but what you can do for your country."

Gene Tierney met the handsome John F. Kennedy, a young World War II veteran, when he was visiting the set of *Dragonwyck* in 1946. They began a romance that ended the following year after Kennedy told her he could never marry her because of his political ambitions and his need to be seen as a proper Catholic who did not marry divorcees. She was broken-hearted for quite some time but sent Kennedy a note of congratulations on his 1960 victory in the presidential election.

In September 1947, a spell of indolence was upon Jack. He became ill in London and was diagnosed at the London Clinic with Addison's disease, a rare endocrine disorder. Davis estimated that Kennedy would die of this within a year. His family insisted he be sent home, but his condition deteriorated while crossing the Atlantic Ocean and a priest was summoned to perform last rites. He held on until he arrived home where doctors saved his life.

Former Vice President Dick Cheney and his longtime cardiologist, Dr. Jonathan Reiner, wrote the 2013 book *Heart: An American Medical Odyssey* about Cheney's thirty-five-year battle with heart disease and the incredible medical breakthroughs that have changed cardiac care over the last four decades. Kennedy and his doctors could have written a book about how the treatment of Addison's diseases kept changing through John Kennedy's lifetime, so that he was always just a step away from death but survived thanks to his physicians and new medical discoveries.

In 1951, John was on a trip in Asia with brother Robert when he suffered a recurrence of his Addison's disease in Tokyo. His temperature surged to 105.8 degrees. He became delirious and then comatose. Those around him did not think we would survive so a priest was called in to deliver last rites. Robert Kennedy found a way to transport John to a military hospital in Okinawa. They saved John's life and the 34-year-old slowly convalesced until he was well enough to travel back home.[6]

In 1954, two years after being elected to the U.S. Senate, Kennedy underwent surgery to fuse his spinal disks. It was a risky operation, but Jack was told that if he didn't have surgery, he might be confined to a wheelchair for life. After the operation, he developed a urinary tract infection that became profoundly serious due to his Addison's disease. His temperature again spiked so high that he fell into a coma and was not expected to live through the night. A priest was called to administer the last rights. Fortunately, he managed to pull through and spent five months recovering.[7]

John Kennedy met Jacqueline Bouvier when she interviewed him as a reporter for the *Washington Times-Herald*. Perhaps he recalled his relationship with reporter Inga Arvad. They announced their engagement on June 24, 1953. They married on September 12, 1953, and honeymooned in Acapulco and Santa Barbara, California. But John was his father's son and on August 23, 1956, Jackie delivered a stillborn daughter while he yachted in the Mediterraneum with a mistress.[8]

In 1958, Jacqueline Kennedy's friend, Adele Astaire Douglass (sister of Fred Astaire) introduced Jackie to Bunny Mellon. The wealthy woman was 19 years older than Jackie, but they became longtime friends and Bunny helped her create her life after the Kennedy assassination. Bunny Mellon, of the Mellon banking magnate, was the style icon who designed the White House Rose Garden for the Kennedys.⁹

On September 26, 1960, John Kennedy was running for president and was to debate Richard Nixon. A week earlier, Kennedy's Harvard classmate investment banker Charles "Chuck" Spalding described having used injections by Dr. Max Jacobson when he sought relief from exhaustion. Spalding told Kennedy, "I went over the top of the building. I felt wonderful, full of energy, capable of doing just about anything. I didn't know exactly what he was giving me, but it was a magic potion." Kennedy had also heard from his *Life Magazine* photographer Mark Shaw who covered Kennedy's campaign that he was greatly energized after seeing Jacobson.¹⁰

Kennedy asked Spalding to set up an appointment. John eluded his security detail and Secret Service men to see Jacobson one afternoon in September 1960. His arrival was expected, and he was served with courtesy and dispatch. He told Jacobson that the grind of campaigning left him tired and weak. Kennedy allowed Jacobson to give him a shot and his muscle weakness immediately disappeared. Jacobson gave Kennedy a bottle of vitamin drops to be taken orally and he departed.¹¹

Kennedy met secretly with Jacobson a few minutes just before he took the stage for the debate. The senator was complaining of his lethargic voice and Jacobson injected his throat pumping methamphetamine into his voice box. That allowed Kennedy to debate without muscle pain and tension. Nixon, who decided to wear no makeup for television, began to sweat profusely and looked very tense. These debates made all the difference about who was elected president thus Kennedy valued Max Jacobson highly.

John Kennedy wanted Max to move to Washington and give up his New York practice. The doctor declined so Kennedy's photographer, Mark Shaw, piloted his own Cessna and flew Jacobson to the Kennedys whenever needed. Jacobson carried his medical supplies in a briefcase for such trips.[12]

Kennedy and Jacobson set up a secret code. Whenever the president wanted to see Jacobson, he or his staff were to call Jacobson's office and say, "There is a call from Mrs. Dunn." Then, Jacobson made himself available when and where a treatment was needed. As the Secret Service became aware of Dr. Jacobson's treatments, and often knew when the president was being whisked away to see "Dr. Feelgood."

The fiasco of the Bay of Pigs invasion plunged Kennedy into deep humiliation. By April 19, 1961, the Cuban government had captured or killed the invading exiles. Kennedy was forced to negotiate for the release of the 1,189 survivors. The stress and humiliation were so deep that Press secretary Pierre Salinger found him weeping in his room on that day.[13]

One day in May 1961, Dr. Jacobson was asked to fly to Palm Beach where the first family was vacationing. Upon arrival, John said Jackie was suffering from depression after giving birth to their son, John Jr. in November. That made the president wonder if she could accompany him on his upcoming trip to Europe where she was to converse in French with General Charles De Gaulle and his wife. The president wanted the doctor to pep her up and called her condition "post-partum depression."

However, Jacqueline may have been depressed over the many affairs her husband was having. It was only four months since taking office and he began an affair during his first month at the White House with 19-year-old intern Mimi Alford according to her memoir *Once Upon a Secret: My Affair with John F. Kennedy and its Aftermath*. In addition, John had urged Jacqueline Kennedy to hire Pamela Turnure as her press secretary, since she had been his secretary when he was a senator. She did so and may have known of their two-year affair. That was described in *The Kennedy Half-Century* by Larry J. Sabato.

Mrs. Kennedy probably did not describe John's affairs to Dr. Jacobson. After he gave her a shot, her mood changed completely. Ten days later, he was summoned to treat her again. After receiving an injection, she told the doctor her husband wanted to see him. John had injured his back during a tree-planting ceremony in Canada and needed an injection.

The president's doctor, Janet Travell had been injecting the anesthetic procaine into his back several times a day. That was in addition to corticosteroids for his Addison's disease. Combining medicines and doctors without their knowledge of what each was doing risked life and limb.

Facial and bodily changes had begun to appear on John Kennedy's body. Steroids cause a flushed countenance and a full rounded face, and fat deposits between the shoulders ("buffalo hump") caused by fluid retention in the tissues. Other side effects include euphoria, agitation, nightmares, hallucinations, and even paranoia. By 1961, photographers noticed the pudginess of Kennedy's face which doctors had already noted. He had a year-round tan, often commented upon by the press, but it came from extra pigmentation of the skin stemming from his Addison's disease. His full head of hair of chestnut brown color also came from Addison's disease and the medication and steroids he was taking.[14]

Jack was hobbling about on crutches and in a week would fly to Europe to meet Khrushchev after De Gaulle. He did not want to appear weak or inadequate after his humiliation over the defeat at the Bay of Pigs six weeks earlier, when Fidel Castro crushed the CIA-backed invasion of Cuba. Jacobson gave him an injection and he was immediately able to walk across the room without crutches. He asked Jacobson to accompany him to the summit in Europe.

A week later, Kennedy had Dr. Jacobson give him an injection aboard Air Force One and had the doctor fly on Air France with nobody else on the plane chartered by the White House. That was surely an outrageous use of taxpayers' money, but he wanted to shield his injections from public attention.

In France, Jacobson injected the president and his wife for conversations with Charles De Gaulle. On June 1, 1961, Jackie was the star of the evening at a state dinner in Versailles, where she spoke fluent French with De Gaulle and his wife. That night, John soaked his back in a giant gold-plated bathtub in the "King's Chamber" of a nineteenth-century palace on the Quai d'Orsay. He received another injection from Jacobson that evening. Mr. and Mrs. Kennedy both received injections when they prepared to meet Queen Elizabeth II in that same trip.[15]

Perhaps Nikita Khrushchev had spies who told him of Kennedy's use of stimulants. Shortly before this trip, Dr. Jacobson's office had been ransacked by the KGB so Kennedy's addiction may have been known. Thusly, Khrushchev arrived to meet Kennedy much later than the original time set for their meeting in Vienna on June 3-4,

1961.[16] The drug was wearing off and the president felt suddenly out of sorts with heavy eyelids and a feverish disposition. He murmured a word with his blurry tongue.

Kennedy's debilitating weakness and his drug addiction gave Khruschev a decided advantage in negotiations. Thus, Nikita's delay left Kennedy in no condition for the important things they were to discuss. Mr. Khrushchev insulted the president, and the president could say little to defend himself or his actions.

Kennedy got into futile debates about communism. Khrushchev then declared that he would sign an agreement to divide Berlin and deny access. He promised to respond with force if the United States challenged the USSR on that issue. Kennedy reacted by saying, "Then, Mr. Chairman, there will be war. It will be a cold winter."

John Kennedy was not smart enough to change his behavior and give up these chemicals. The consequences of his bad experience with Khrushchev did not rouse him to action. Nothing of that sort took place. He was powerless to tear himself away from addictive methamphetamine. If we are under the advice of those who have no understanding (like Dr. Feelgood) we destroy our health. Will life be worth living if that higher part of man be destroyed?

John Kennedy was very reckless in his responsibilities as a president. He was also very reckless in his love affairs which included Judith Campbell Exner, whom he knew was also seeing mob boss Sam Giancana. That man had worked with Al Capone on his way up the ladder to run illegal gambling operations in Chicago.

Exner was invited to Las Vegas by Frank Sinatra as part of the rat-pack Hollywood crowd. On February 7, 1960, she was introduced to presidential candidate John Kennedy in Dean Martin's hotel suite. Her affair with Kennedy began in March 1960, in New York.

In her autobiography, she denied being a go-between but admitted passing messages to Giancana from entertainers like Jerry Lewis and Eddie Fisher. She became a patient of Dr. Max Jacobson. Since she was under close observation by the FBI, at J. Edgar Hoover's request Kennedy finally dropped her.[17]

Kennedy's White House physician, Janet Travell, was aware of John's search for pain killers. She knew of some treatment by others but not specifics. However, in November 1961, Dr. Cohen, Kennedy's endocrinologist for the last five years wrote this note to the president:

> You cannot be permitted to receive therapy from irresponsible doctors like M.J. who by forms of stimulating injections offer some temporary help to neurotic or mentally ill individuals... this therapy conditions one's needs almost like a narcotic and is not for responsible individuals who at any split second may have to decide the fate of the universe.[18]

Now, important doctors and men were telling Kennedy that police ought to condemn his drugs.

White House physician Janet Travell had tried to help Kennedy. She found that he had one leg shorter than the other and had a lift made to insert in his left shoe so he could walk more evenly. She recommended the rocking chair which helped relieve discomfort and relaxed him. Other doctors criticized her overuse of procaine for his back pain, and overuse of penicillin. That antibiotic can induce a fatal allergic reaction or can become ineffective with overuse.

Although Kennedy had many infections that responded to penicillin, his main use was to prevent venereal disease. He was like so many men who walked in the door of their doctor's office and announced, "I need a shot of penicillin." They did not even have to say why. Chlamydia, gonorrhea, and syphilis are caused by bacteria that usually respond to penicillin or other strong antibiotics with a single injection.

In June 1962, Kennedy's brother Bobby, the U.S. attorney general, grew so suspicious of Jacobson that he sent a sample of his formula to the FBI to learn what was in it. When he found out it contained amphetamines, he urged his brother not to use it. JFK told him flat out, "I don't care if it's horse piss. It makes me feel good. It works." John Kennedy's corruption lay in his choice of gratifications.

The presidents' wants were supplied. By May 1962, Jacobson had visited the White House 34 times to give the president injection boosts for his struggles.[19]

John Kennedy owned an apartment at the Carlyle Hotel for ten years in New York City's upper east side. It was known as "the New York White House" during his administration. Dr. Jacobson sometimes was sent there and on July 15, 1962, the injection of amphetamines was apparently too high a dose. He went into the living room where the staff were waiting. He started stripping off his clothes and danced around the room naked.

First, his staff men were amused. He was completely naked, on the verge of paranoia thinking his people were against him by trying to restrain him. But he was feeling so free of pain that he almost wanted to perform gymnastic acts as he ran out the door into the hallway. He began running from door to door looking for Mimi Alford, the young aide he had seduced early in his administration. She was waiting in a room at the end of the hall where they were to have a fling.

His staff grabbed him and drug him back into his room as he screamed. They pondered whether they should put the president in a straitjacket. They called prominent New York psychiatrist Lawrence Hatterer who came quickly and recognized the psychotic symptoms. He gave the president an anti-psychotic medicine and within minutes, he returned to more normal behavior.[20]

In addition, John was being given steroids that enhanced the sex drive. England's Prime Minister Harold Macmillan saw some of Kennedy's lovers hiding nearby on their visits and Kennedy confided that if he did not have sex daily, he got a headache.[21]

On February 22, 1963, Mrs. Kennedy called her Secret Service agent Clint Hill with an unusual request. The president announced that he would put his White House staff to a 50-mile walking test expecting to kick-start a national fitness campaign. Mrs. Kennedy told Clint that her brother-in-law Stash Radziwill and Chuck Spalding were going to begin the hike that night. She wanted Clint to be there to ensure that things were okay. She, about three months pregnant, and the president were going to check on the hike from time to time, and Dr. Max Jacobson was to be there for medical help.

Clint reluctantly agreed because he had no time to get other shoes than his dress shoes. Big blisters resulted after several hours. Some walkers took oxygen administered by Jacobson. Photographer Mark Shaw took pictures of the participants, the Kennedys, and the doctor. He published them before he died of amphetamine poisoning given him by Dr. Jacobson. Clint Hill subsequently wrote of this in *Mrs. Kennedy and Me* published in 2012 by Simon and Schuster.[22]

On August 7, 1963, Jacqueline Kennedy gave birth to little Patrick who died the next day. The Kennedys mourned together. Jacqueline could not attend Patrick's funeral because she was recovering from a C-section. So, John attended and took his St. Chrisopher medal from his wallet and placed it in the casket. He then asked White House physician Janet Travell to go with Jackie to Palm Beach to help her recover.[23]

When Jackie learned that John had buried his medal with Patrick, she had a new one made for him. At the president's funeral three months later, Jacqueline was standing by Bobby Kennedy next to the president's casket. She put some items and scribbles from little John and Caroline in the casket. Robert saw that and pulled his own St. Christopher's medal out of his wallet to drop into the casket as well. It had been a gift from his wife, Ethel.[24]

On September 20, 1963, President Kennedy made his speech before the United Nations. His speech ended with this phrase: "Let us take our stand here in this assembly of nations... and move this world to a just and lasting peace." John Kennedy had laryngitis the night before, and had Jacobson inject him at the Carlisle Hotel. The talk went well, and the president thanked him at a reception following the speech.

Dr. Hans Kraus who treated the president's back pain had also hear of Kennedy's treatment by Jacobson and said in December 1962: "If I ever heard he took another shot,

I'd make sure it was known. No President with his finger on the red button has any business taking stuff like that."[25] So many people close to the president saw what he was doing and tried to stop him, but he was living the good life. He was the most important man in the United States, and in the world according to many.

At the end of John Kennedy's life, he was having a glorious moment riding in a limousine as Texas Governor John Connally's wife Nellie said, "Mr. President, you can't say Dallas doesn't love you." Those were the last words John Kennedy ever heard.

From the emergency room at Parkland Hospital, Jacqueline Kennedy asked that a priest be called to administer last rites to the president. It was the parish of Father Oscar Huber, C.M., who arrived within thirty minutes. A sheet covered the president and Huber stood next to Jacqueline to carry out last rites. He said over President Kennedy words such as "I absolve you from your sins in the name of the Father, and of the Son, and of the Holy Ghost. Amen." Jackie then asked Father Huber to pray for her husband.[26]

Huber explained later in an interview that anointing is to be done before the soul has left the body. Huber said the time of the soul leaving the body might be two to three hours after a sudden death, thus last rites could guarantee salvation if the deceased had sorrow for his sins. Father Huber thought that John Kennedy was a good man from what he had read and would have sorrow for his sins. Father Huber donated that interview some months after Kennedy's death to the JFK Library.[27]

As we all know, Jacqueline Kennedy married Aristotle Onassis. She remained friends with Chuck Spalding who had introduced John Kennedy to Max Jacobson just before the Kennedy-Nixon debates. On May 28, 1973, some ten years after the Kennedy assassination, Max Jacobson got a call from Spalding who said he urgently needed to meet. The next day, the doctor was surprised to find Jacqueline Onassis waiting for him. Jacobson was to speak with a panel reviewing his license in two more days. Through the years, Jacobson had bragged about treating the president, and wore off his PT-109 tie clasp as a badge of honor given him by President Kennedy.

Jackie wanted to know what he would say if asked about the White House. He assured her that there was no reason for concern. He mentioned that he had never taken money from Kennedy but was concerned about the hearing and had spent $35,000 on legal fees. She told him, "You don't have anything to worry about," suggesting that she might finance his legal help. He was discreet and details about treatment of the Kennedys did not emerge for many years.[28]

What a strange adventure Jacqueline had shared with John Kennedy. She undoubtedly wondered how her actions would be seen and hoped that she would not be humiliated if news of their drug abuse surfaced. As we all know, Aristotle Onassis was helpful in facing the future with her children. After his death, she had companions, but became ill with non-Hodgkin's lymphoma and died at 64. She was buried next to President John Kennedy.

It seemed that most of Kennedy's physicians wanted what was best for him and for the country. But they were hampered by a patient who sought treatment from doctors on his own and failed to inform them of treatments by others. He did not reveal his medical history to the Navy, or to the public when his health was questioned during the presidential campaign. He did not care that Max Jacobson had no hospital privileges and wrote no prescriptions. Dr. Feelgood made his own medicines in his filthy laboratory with his dirty fingernails touching syringes, and used his drugs which clouded his own mind.

There is no doubt that Kennedy's actions often resulted from his background of suffering. However, his wants for sex and pain relief were like someone saying, "I want what I want when I want it." He gave little thought to serving his country with a clouded mind that might plunge the world into war. He eluded the bagman carrying the satchel of vital communications when he desired a sexual tryst. He cared little about hurting the feelings of those in his life.

President Kennedy, his wife, his friends, and some of his doctors lacked integrity. President Thomas Jefferson said, "God grant that men of principle shall be our principal men." We must hope that future presidents will be more honest and care more for the country they serve. Many believe that the successful whitewash of Kennedy's medical history and health should push the United States to explore how this might be prevented in the future.

Jerrold M. Post 1934-2020) was an American psychiatrist and author. He was an analyst for the Central Intelligence Agency and the founder of the Center for the Analysis of Personality and Political Behavior, and helped found our International Society of Political Psychologists in 1978. Post created several «psychobiography's» of notable individuals during his tenure at the C.I.A. and wrote *Dangerous Charisma* about Donald Trump, predicting that he would not accept election results if he lost.

Post wrote *When Illness Strikes the Leader* in 1995 and discussed John Kennedy and others. He also wrote an article entitled "Substance Abuse" for *The Washington Post* published on January 28, 1990.[29]

Here is an excerpt of that article:

It appears that amphetamine abuse, which had spread to the general population in the 1960s, began in elite groups in the 1940s and '50s. "Celebrity doctors" may have played an important role in first establishing this pattern.

Dr. Max Jacobson had fled Hitler's Germany in 1936 and soon took up medical practice in New York City. Although he had no staff privileges at any hospital after 1946, he acquired a reputation as a doctor for celebrities, among whom he was known as "Doctor Feel-good."...

Among the initial effects of amphetamines which make it attractive to a leader in a crisis are an increase of alertness, lessened fatigue, feelings of well-being and lessened need for sleep. In a crisis, an individual "high" on stimulants may be insufficiently cautious or unduly optimistic. Under sustained stress, some will utilize serially stimulant amphetamine and hypnotic drugs, producing a "high-low" sequence...

Decisions are made without judicious consideration, in impulsive haste. Continued amphetamine use can lead to confusion about time and place, distractibility, vagueness, rambling speech, delusions of persecution, hallucinations and psychologic behavior resembling paranoid schizophrenia...

World leaders operate under unusual stress and often feel entitled to special treatment. Substance abuse by major political leaders is not a private illness. For the leader under the influence of drugs or alcohol... every aspect of his functioning is affected--his perceptions, judgment, decision-making and the balance between his own needs and those of his followers. Especially during crises, when the mighty are high, the lowly should tremble... To put things in a different light, if an officer in the U.S. Air Force were taking any one of these medications, he or she would not even be allowed to talk on the radio to aircraft as supervisor of flying. Kennedy, as commander-in-chief, was supervisor for the entire Air Force.

When John Kennedy became president, he hoped that his health problems would not prevent him from handling the job. By hiding his medical problems, he kept voters from deciding whether they wanted to take a chance on him or not. If the public had known more about him and his medications, would he have even been nominated or elected?

Notes

1. https://www.cbc.ca/radio/undertheinfluence/john-f-kennedy-was-given-last-rites-5-different -times-1.6362855
2. https://www.vanityfair.com/news/2009/03/dietrich-kennedy200803
3. "Kennedy Affair with Spy Suspect Reported" *Los Angeles Times* January 19, 1976., p. B8
4. *Jack Kennedy* by Chris Matthews, 2011, p. 44 and https://warfare historynetwork.com/article/wwii-secrets-the-mysterious-inga-arvad/

5. http://news.google.com/newspaper? Id=3XUbAAAAIBAJ& sjid-kowEAAAAIBAJ&pg=3103,31675&dq=arvad&hl=en
6. https://www.cbc.ca/radio/undertheinfluence/john-f-kennedy-was-given-last-rites-5-diferent-times-1.6362855
7. https://www.cbc.ca/radio/undertheinfluence/john-f-kennedy-was-given-last-rites-5-diferent-times-1.6362855
8. "JFK and Jackie Kennedy's Relationship Timeline" by Nicole Briese for *People Magazine*, July 12, 2023.
9. https://www.townandcountrymag.com/society/money-and-power/a41916235/jackie-kennedy-bunny-mellon-friendship-true-story/
10. https://www.historynet.com/jack-kennedy-dr-feelgood/
11. https://www.historynet.com/jack-kennedy-dr-feelgood/
12. "President Kennedy's Nutrition Physician, Dr. Max Jacobson" by David A. Jeand'Heur and Andrew W Saul published by *Orthomolecular Medicine*.
13. Dallek, Robert. *An Unfinished Life: John F. Kennedy 1917-1963*, Boston: Little, Brown, 2003, p. 366.
14. *Ailing, Aging, Addicted*. Bert E. Park, M.D. The University Press of Kentucky, 1993.
15. https://www.atlanticcouncil.org/content-series/thinking-global/berlin-1961-kennedy-s-dr-feelgood/
16. nypost.com/2013/04/21/the-kennedy-meth/
17. https://www.nytimes.com/1977/06/13/archives/frank-jack-sam-judy.html
18. http://hnn.us/articles/1124.html)
19. https://telemachusunedited.wordpress.com/tag/max-jacobson/
20. "Amphetamines Used by a Physician to Life Moods of Famous Patients" by Boyce Rensberger, Dec. 7, 1972, *The New York Times*, and https://www.nytimes.com/1972/12/04/archives/amphetamines-used-by-a-physician-to-lift-moods-of-famous-patients.html
21. https://nypost.com/2013/11/10/all-the-presidents-women-3/

22. https://clinthillsecretservice.com/2017/02/23/jackie-jfk-50-mile-hike/
23. Oral History Interview with Janet G. Travell on January 20, 1966, in Washington, D.C. by Theodore C. Sorenson for the John F. Kennedy Library [24].\[24] https://historical.ha.com/itm/political/presidential-relics/john-f-kennedy-his-well-used-leather-wallet-and-1959-61-massachusetts-drivers-license/a/6142-48013.s
25. https://www.nytimes.com/2008/05/29/opinion/129jfk.html and https://www.irishcentral.com/roots/history/john-f-kennedy-max-jacobson
26. https://parade.com/232133/parade/priest-who-gave-jfk-his-last-rites-i-assured-mrs-kenedy-i-would-pray-for-the-president/
27. https://www.jfklibrary.org/sites/default/files/archives/JFKOH/Huber%2C%20Oscar%20L/JFKOH-OLH-01/JFKOH-OLH-01-TR.pdf) Source: "The Strange Saga of JFK and the Original 'Dr. Feelgood'" Peter Keating, November 22, 2013.
28. http://nymag.com/intelligencer/2013/11/strange-saga-of-jfk-and-dr-feelgood.html)
29. https://www.washingtonpost.com/archive/opinions/1990/01/28/substance-abuse/e2c9a3da-12a5-4893-908a-3f2b92f19925/

Hedy Lamarr

Hedwig Eva Maria Kiesler (1918-2000) was born in Vienna, Austria. Her Jewish father was a banker, and her mother was a concert pianist. She won a beauty contest at twelve and starred in a silent movie called *Money on the Street* in 1930. Her next movie was produced by Max Reinhardt called *The Trunks of Mr. O.F.*, 1931, starring Walter Abel and Peter Lorre. At age eighteen, she was given the lead role in *Ecstasy*, playing the neglected young wife and an older man. Scenes of nudity and her face during orgasm were highlighted. The film was banned in many places and caused her some embarrassment later.

In addition to her beauty, she developed an interest in science. From an early age, she strolled with her father who described inventions and technology to her. She came to appreciate how to talk to men. Her first marriage was at 18 to wealthy 33-year-old Friedrich Mandl, an Austrian military arms merchant and manufacturer. He was close to Italian fascist leader Benito Mussolini, and later Adolf Hitler.

She took acting classes, but her husband prevented her from continuing her acting career. She disliked how he controlled her life. Before two years of marriage had passed, she took some jewels and disguised herself as a maid and fled to Paris. She divorced while in France. Looking for a way to appear in American movies, she saw news that Louis B. Mayer, head of MGM studio, was in Europe scouting for European talent. Unable to get a satisfactory appointment with him, she sailed to America on the ship he was on.

He spent time with her aboard and was impressed. He signed her to a contract for $500 a week by the time they arrived in the United States. She changed her name to Hedy Lamarr, at the suggestion of his wife, in homage to silent film star Barbara La Marr. Mayer described her as the "world's most beautiful woman."

She made movies with King Vidor, as well, and he was delighted when Hedy kissed him at the conclusion of one of their two movies, *H. M. Pulham, Esq.* in 1941.[1] Earlier, he had thought, "How dare you smile like that. No one is allowed to smile like that!"

She met George Antheil, American composer and pianist, at a party in early 1942. They began talking about how radio-controlled torpedoes being used at that time in WWII were easily jammed and sent off course. Together with Antheil, who used player piano rolls, they produced the idea of using an encrypted frequency-hopping signal to avoid jamming. The device was based on the idea of a piano roll that randomly changed the signal sent between the control center and torpedo at short bursts within a range of 88 frequencies on the spectrum, corresponding to the 88 black and white keys on a piano keyboard.

They worked very hard to get the specifications right. They toiled over the patent requirements. Then when it was approved, they were triumphant in possession of the truth of their work at last.

Lamarr and Antheil obtained a joint patent in 1942 for this torpedo with a radio-guidance system. The military never picked up the idea, but her achievements were finally recognized in 1997 when she received a "Pioneer Award" from the Electronic Frontier Foundation. In fact, their idea was a precursor to spread-spectrum technology—or digital wireless communications—that gives us wireless phones, GPS and Wi-fi today. Antheil died in 1959 and was quickly forgotten. Lamarr got a star on the Hollywood Walk of Fame. Posthumously, both were inducted into the National Inventors Hall of Fame in 2014.

Hedy wrote an autobiography entitled *Ecstasy and Me* in 1970. After Mandel, she was married to Gene Markey 1939-1941, actor John Loder 1943-1947, Teddy Stauffer 1951-1952, W. Howard Lee 1953-1960 who later married actress Gene Tierney, and Lewis J. Boises 1963-1965. She and handsome British star Loder starred in 1947 *Dishonored Lady* and had three children during their brief marriage.

Here are a few quotations in Lamar movies. From 1938 *Algiers,* her co-star was Charles Boyer as Pepe Le Moko and she was Gaby:

Boyer: What did you do before?
Lamarr: Before what?
Boyer: Before the jewels.
Lamarr: I wanted them.
In 1947 *Dishonored Lady*, Lamarr co-starred with husband/costar John Loder:
Loder: Say, women are supposed to scream. Are you afraid of mice?
Lamarr: No, but next time I'll scream.

After some pictures, she went to work under Cecil B. DeMille in *Samson and Delilah*. That turned out to be one of her biggest hits. DeMille was a believer in Max Jacobson's liquid vitamin injections. Sadly, Hedy developed a 25-year habit of using those amphetamine-laced concoctions. They played a role in her gradual deterioration.

Lamarr was also interested in maintaining her looks through plastic surgery. She shared ideas with her physicians about how this might be done best. It was as if she wanted to be forever crystallized, like Snow White asleep in her glass coffin. Unfortunately, some of her ideas led to problems so that her beautiful face changed over the years. Toward the end, she thought it best to admit once and for all that her face became rather homely. But thankfully the sun shines with the same penetrating clarity upon the lovely and the commonplace.

She became a loner, something like Greta Garbo, because she did not want to be seen. She could talk for hours by phone with people who could remember her beauty. She was arrested in 1966 and 1991 for stealing small items from stores. Charges were dropped when she was recognized as the great actress and promised not to do it again.

In a curious way, she gained fame from a Mel Brooks 1974 movie called *Blazing Saddles* with a character named Hedley Lamarr, which was almost her name. She sued the studio, and settled out of court for an undetermined amount which satisfied her, plus an apology.

A movie about her life was written by Esther Saks and financed by actress Susan Sarandon entitled *Bombshell* in 2017.[2]

Notes

1. *A Tree Is a Tree* by King Vidor, Llongmans, Green and Co., 1954 published next door to author Cheney's travel agency office in London on Clifford Street. The author ran a travel agency called Study Abroad, Inc. for tourists to visit the British Isles in 1957-59 and officed in London.
2. jewcy.com/arts-and-culture/bombshell-hedy-lamarr-story/

Alan Jay Lerner

Alan Jay Lerner (1918-1986) was the son of Edith and Joseph Lerner, the brother of Samuel Lerner, owner of the Lerner dress shops. Alan Lerner's cousin was TV game show panelist Henry Morgan. Alan was a classmate of John F. Kennedy at Choate where they worked together on the yearbook staff. Like Cole Porter at Yale and Richard Rodgers at Colombia, Lerner's career began with the Harvard Hasty Pudding musicals.

While attending Harvard in 1936 and 1937, Alan lost an eye due to a boxing accident, thus he did not serve in WWII. He wrote radio scripts for the popular *Your Hit Parade* show. He met Austrian composer Frederick Lowe, who was looking for a partner in 1942. They collaborated to produce a musical that ran on Broadway for several weeks in 1943. They created music and song to charm the souls of men and women for many years.

Their first big hit was 1947 romantic fantasy set in the mystical Scottish village of *Brigadoon*. That was followed by 1951 *Paint Your Wagon* which included the song "They Call the Wind Mariah." He also did the screenplay for *An American in Paris* directed by Vincente Minnelli, who would later join Lerner and Loewe for *Gigi*.

They did *My Fair Lady* in 1956, adapting George Bernand Shaw's *Pygmalion*. The characters of Henry Higgins and Eliza Doolittle were played by Rex Harrison and Julie Andrews in the movie. Lerner was hospitalized for bleeding ulcers when they worked on *Camelot* in 1960. Loewe retired and Lerner went on to make other musicals. Strangely due to a comment by Jacqueline after the assassination of President Kennedy, *Camelot* became a great hit with audiences.

During the filming of the 1970 *On a Clear Day You Can See Forever*, Dr. Max Jacobson was a guest on the yacht of lyricist Alan Jay Lerner. The doctor injected Lerner and other members of the cast and crew with a cocktail of drugs that allowed them to work around the clock. That movie was about a woman who had been reincarnated, starring Barbara Streisand, Yves Montand, Bob Newhart, Jack Nicholson, and was directed by Vincente Minnelli.[1]

For nearly twenty years, Lerner was addicted to amphetamines administered by Dr. Max Jacobson and his injections of "vitamins with enzymes."[2]

Lerner was married eight times and had four children. Love and women were so important to Lerner that he didn't want them to be standardized. Romance thrilled him. Women were bowled over by the extent of his drug use and his clouded mind that could produce such musical hits.

Near the time of his death, he wanted to finish a last project because he was losing his memory and had developed metastatic lung cancer. He walked about with a bent head in which strains of music were hammered out with rhymes anew. He was not feeling well and had to struggle against a sense of futility and hopelessness. He died in 1986 of lung cancer at age 67, married to actress Liz Robertson, some 36 years younger than he. Lerner owed IRS over a million dollars in back taxes and was unable to pay for his final medical expenses. Another life left in ruins by the seemingly helpful Dr. Max Jacobson. On a clear day, Alan Lerner could not see forever.

Notes

1. https://www.sarasotamagazine.com/arts-and-entertainment/2011/11/this-way-to-broadway)
2. http://www.nysuhn.com/out-and-about/dr-feelgood/20251/

Mickey Mantle

Mickey Mantle (1931-1995) was an American baseball player born in Oklahoma. His father was a baseball player who wanted a son to become one. Mickey went through high school sports concentrating on himself. He had no responsibilities and was popular with boys and girls. He was a carefree youth who loved the spotlight.

After high school, he was offered a football scholarship by the University of Oklahoma. He declined it at his father's request. Mickey sustained an injury in football and developed osteomyelitis, an infectious disease, that was treated with the new antibiotic, penicillin. That reduced the infection and saved his leg from amputation. That infection in his left leg gave him a 4-F deferment during the Korean War. He disliked the negative publicity about a physical flaw in his body.

He married Merlyn Johnson in 1951 and they had four sons.

He was selected by the Yankees but had to show people that despite being disqualified to serve in the military, he was a tough guy. After a brief slump, he was sent to the Kansas City Blues. However, he went on to the Yankees and impressed everyone in the early 1950s. His career was on the rise, and everything seemed to be going his way.

His wild life of drinking began to catch up with him and by 1960, he was a very heavy alcoholic. In September 1961 Mantle was feeling poorly. On an airplane September 24, 1961, the returning players and sportscasters shared comments with each other. Mantle was suffering from a cold and upper respiratory infection. He chatted about his lethargy with Mel Allen, known as the Voice of the

New York Yankees. Mickey wanted to get back in good shape because he was inspired by the records of other Yankee players who were Babe Ruth, Lou Gehrig, and Joe DiMaggio. He and teammate Roger Maris set out to beat Babe Ruth's record of sixty homeruns.

Mel Allen commented that his doctor, Max Jacobson, could help Mickey feel better. Mel made an appointment for Mantle and upon arrival, Max Jacobson told him to pull down his pants. He did so and the syringe went into his hip and apparently hit the bone. Mantle felt terrible pain. He noted that the doctor's office seemed dirty, and thought the doctor used a bad needle.[1]

The hip injection site was painful, bled freely, but Mantle tried to be tough and simply covered it with bandages. But the longer he walked, the more he was tortured. The blood continued to pour out with movement, so he was hitting the ball, getting to first base, and another player would run the other bases for him.

Jane Leavey wrote her 2010 Mantle biography entitled *The Last Boy* describing the abscess at the injection site. This wound ended his chance at the home run record, as well as threatening Mantle's career. He suffered agonies at the thought of failure. She described how Jacobson's amphetamines and other drugs were producing addiction, withdrawal symptoms, and ruining the lives of other patients as well as his.

He was the American League Most Valuable Player three times and was inducted into the Baseball Hall of Fame in 1974. Had he had fallen in love with himself, the one person he could never possess?

Mickey next learned that he had liver cancer due to cirrhosis caused by his heavy drinking. His career fizzled out. He knew there was something not quite right about his career. He began to tell young people not to use him as a role model because despite treatment at the Betty Ford Center for alcohol rehabilitation, he felt he was not a good role model for young fellows. His biography in *The Last Boy* is an informative and haunting book.

Note

1. https://www.grunge.com/852746/how-the-real-dr-feelgood-prevented-possible-baseball-history/

Johnny Mathis

John Mathis was born in Gilmer, Texas, in 1935, to parents who were domestic cooks, but his father had been a vaudeville singer and pianist. His family moved to San Francisco when Johnny was five, and his parents encouraged him to sing and do sports. He was a star athlete as a high jumper and basketball player. In 1954, he attended college on an athletic scholarship intending to be a physical education teacher.

However, afternoon jam sessions turned into regular singing, and he recorded songs beginning in 1955. He appeared on *The Ed Sullivan Show* in 1957, cut records, and was in occasional movies. His velvety voice, good looks, and gentlemanly demeanor won him countless fans. He gradually became a millionaire and tried to protect his name and reputation.

He became a homosexual and covered that up for years until 1982. He sang for royalty like Prince Charles and Princess Diana and for presidents Reagan and Clinton. His number one hit was "Chances Are" recorded when he was 23. "When a Child Is Born" has been a Christmas favorite which went to Number One in 1976. His music became the soundtrack for a few movies such as *Goodfellas* and *Mad Men*.

He attended a wedding reception with Ronald and Nancy Reagan. He was conversing with Nancy while slurping down champagne and she questioned him. She was known to tell youth "Just say no" when someone offered drugs to them during Reagan's term of office.

Mathis confessed that he could not stop drinking. She sent him to Have de Grace in Maryland which was run by Jesuit priests. He said, "I had three weeks of finding out why I drank, how I could stop. And it was the greatest thing that ever happened to me in my life."[1]

He also went to Dr. Max Jacobson and said this about that treatment in a Media interview on January 6, 2015:

> I went to see him because I was doing five shows a night at the Copacabana in New York and got laryngitis. Everyone on Broadway went to him and so did the Kennedys. He gave me vitamin shots which brought my voice back beautifully but left me with a drug addiction. It was very traumatic, but I just had to stop. I also drank too much, only champagne, and I never thought too much about it until I was talking to Nancy Reagan at a reception, and she asked if I always drank so much. I said yes and she said, 'Well, don't you think it's bad for you?' and I said, 'Yes, but I don't know how to stop.' The next thing I know she collared the Chief of Staff and I'm on a plane to a rehab facility. I stayed three weeks, and I haven't drunk since. That was thirty years ago.

He was very embarrassed to be a drug addict.[2] Although 87-year-old singer Johnny Mathis was a bit hunched over, he was still performing to big audiences in 2023 as can be seen on *YouTube*. Wisdom was achieved by taking responsibility for changing his behavior and withstanding temptation.

Notes

1. https://www.foxnews.com/entertainment/johnny-mathis-is-forever-grateful-to-nancy-reagan.print
2. https://mediainterviews.wordpress.com/2015/01/06/johnny-mathis-realising-i-was-a-drug-addict-was-so-traumatic/

Liza Minnelli

Liza Minnelli was the daughter of singer and actress Judy Garland and movie director Vincente Minnelli born in 1946. She became an actress, singer, dancer, and choreographer. Although she did not exactly follow in the footsteps of her mother, the apple doesn't fall far from the tree.

She was uncredited as a child in 1949 *In the Good Old Summertime*, 1954 *The Long, Long Trailer*, and 1968 *The Odd Couple*. She appeared in 1969 *The Sterile Cuckoo*, 1970 *Tell Me That You Love Me Junie Moon*, 1972 *Cabaret* directed by Bob Fosse, 1974 *That's Entertainment*, 1976 *Silent Movie*, and 1976 *A Matter of Time* starring Ingrid Bergman and directed by her father, Vincente Minnelli.

Here is some dialogue by Liza from *Cabaret* with actor Michael York:

> York: You're American.
> Minnelli: Oh, God, how depressing! You're meant to think I'm an international woman of mystery. I'm working on it like mad.

Here is dialogue by Liza in *A Matter of Time* with Ingrid Bergman as the Contessa.

> Bergman: Now, you look as you should. You may go now.
> Minnelli: Oh, Contessa, thank you.
> Bergman: Oh, don't thank me. I'm merely teaching myself to grow old in the right way. I'll wish you as much happiness, as much suffering in your life as I've had in mine. Go along now.

Liza was sometimes asked to take sides supporting either her mother or her father in one issue or another. She continually said things like, "I don't take sides," or "I am on the side of truth." She took her father's side in his poignant tale and cast of 1976, Liza *A Matter of Time*.

That movie was a musical fantasy directed by her father starring Charles Boyer, Ingrid Bergman, Ingrid's daughter Isabella Rossellini, and Tina Aumont, daughter of Jean-Pierre Aumont and Dominican actress Maria Montez. This was the third and last time that Bergman and Boyer starred together, having been in *Gaslight* and *Arch of Triumph* earlier. In her autobiography, she called him the "smartest" actor she knew.

This movie contained the George Gershwin song "Do It Again," and while the movie was no big hit, it was sentimental as we saw some of these actors for the last time. In the 1970s, Charles Boyer went for a health check-up and suggested his wife of 44 years, English actress Pat Paterson go also. Unbeknownst to Pat, she was diagnosed with inoperable colon and liver cancer with less than a year to live.

Boyer did not tell her but moved them to Paradise Valley near Scottsdale, Arizona, supposedly for his health. He read constantly to his wife as she became sicker. He refused to let nurses take care of her. She died at age 67 in 1978 as he held her hand. Their son had committed suicide at age 21. Two days after Pat died, Charles visited friends and took an overdose of Seconal sleeping pills. He was found and taken to a Phoenix hospital but died and was buried next to his son and wife.

Liza also starred in 1977 *New York New York,* 1981 *Arthur,* 1985 *That's Dancing* and other movies. She was on television in many specials. She has sung many songs, but her signature song was "New York New York."

Minnelli returned to Broadway in 1997 replacing Julie Andrews in the musical *Victor/Victoria*. However, she developed viral encephalitis in 2000 and was very ill. She had to take vocal and dance lessons to return to her former work, with the aid of friends.[1]

Kay Thompson had been given free housing at the Plaza Hotel in New York City for nearly twenty years because she had written books about Eloise, a child who roamed the Plaza. However, when Thompson stopped writing, the hotel evicted her in 1973. Liza allowed Kay to live with her rent-free until Thompson died in 1998.

In 2007, Liza was working on an album in tribute to Kay Thompson whom Judy Garland chose as Liza's godmother. Liza, Judy, and many others were trained by Thompson to sing big hits with enthusiasm and showmanship. When Kay became addicted to Max Jacobson's amphetamine-laced vitamin injections, Liza shared that usage with her for some time.

Liza was a surprise guest at the 2022 94th Academy Awards ceremony. She presented the Best Picture award along with Lady Gaga. Liza was in a wheelchair and fumbled with the papers of the nominees, but she was assisted by Lady Gaga. She looked quite upbeat when *CODA* about deaf people won the Best Picture award.

During her lifetime, Minnelli served on the board of charities and non-profits. She dedicated much time to The Foundation for AIDS Research founded by Elizabeth Taylor. She said in 2007 that such an organization was important because she had lost so many friends to AIDS.

Note

1. https://www.theguardian.com/music/2008/may/04/popandrock)

Christopher Plummer

Arthur Christopher Plummer (1929-2021) was born in Toronto, Canada, to a stockbroker and his wife who worked as a secretary at McGill University. Plummer's second cousin was British actor Nigel Bruce who portrayed Doctor Watson to Basil Rathbone's Sherlock Holmes movies. Plummer's parents separated shortly after his birth, and he grew up with his mother in Quebec becoming fluent in English and French. He began acting in high school and then did stage work in Ottawa with apprenticing actor William Shatner who became his lifelong friend.

Plummer acted in Canada, England, and the United States in movies as well as television. His breakthrough role was Captain Von Trapp with Julie Andrews in 1965 *The Sound of Music*. He went on to star in other movies such as 1964 *The Fall of the Roman Empire,* 1979 *Hanover Street,* 2001 *A Beautiful Mind,* 2011 *The Captains* written and directed by William Shatner, 2011 *The Girl with the Dragon Tattoo* and 2019 *Knives Out.*

Here is a bit of dialogue from *Hanover Street* between Christopher Plummer and Harrison Ford:

> Plummer: How far do you think we've gone?
> Ford: How am I supposed to know? You're the god damn spy, not me. Don't you guys have a magic manual or something that teaches you all that stuff?
> Plummer: Yes, we do.
> Ford: Did you ever read it?
> Plummer: I helped write it.

Plummer received an Academy Award for Best Supporting Actor in 2011, two Tony awards, a BAFTA Award, and other awards. Plummer married actress Tammy Grimes from 1956 to 1960, journalist Patricia Lewis from 1962 to 1967 and actress Elaine Taylor in 1970. He wrote a memoir entitled *In Spite of Myself*, published by Alfred A. Knopf in 2008. He described his experience with Dr. Max Jacobson in his memoir on pages 233-235:

> Dr. Max Jacobson, or "Miracle Max" as he was more commonly known, was a cross between Conrad Veidt and Martin Borman. His reputation for getting people who were near death's door back on their feet in a manner of seconds was the talk of the town. This had earned him his nickname. Opera stars who had lost their voices, politicians who had lost their nerve, dancers, actors, athletes, all plaintively knocked on his door begging for the "cure." He was also society's darling—they called him "Dr. Feelgood..."
>
> Later President Kennedy would make him part of the White House inner circle as his private saviour, summoning him for treatment whenever or wherever he felt pain or flagging energy...
>
> "Vell? Vat happent to you?" This darkly sinister man shouted at me. I felt I was in *the cabinet of Dr. Caligari.*
>
> "I put my knee out, Doctor."

"I know vat you dit. I asked you vat happen?!"

I told him the whole grisly story, adding that I had to perform the next day... He was out of the room in a flash. He reappeared brandishing two long thin sticks with cotton, one soaked in some liquid, the other covered with white powder. He stuck them both so far up my nose I heard it crack.

"But Doctor Jacobson, it's my knee, not my nose!"

"Shaddup undt mindt your own business," he retorted as he shot me at least six times around the knee area.

"Now stand up on your feet undt get outta here!"

I didn't walk, I leapt. I was Superman. True to his name, Miracle Max had done me proud.

Conscience reproached Plummer as if he had debauched. It wasn't good to feel so good. It was bad to feel this good. So, Christopher finally escaped from *The Cabinet of Dr. Caligari,* which he had mentioned. That was a silent 1920 German horror film with Conrad Veidt (who played Major Strasser in *Casablanca).* Plummer changed his life, so he no longer had to deal with the German doctor.

Anthony Quinn

Manuel Antonio Rodolfo Quinn Oaxaca (1915-2001) was born in Chihuahua, Mexico to an Irish immigrant father and Mexican mother. His father was reported to have ridden with Mexican revolutionary Pancho Villa, before moving to Los Angeles where he became an assistant cinematographer in a movie studio.[1]

At age 11, he joined the Pentecostals at the International Church of the Foursquare Gospel, founded by Aimee Semple McPherson. He played in the church band while being an apprentice preacher with McPherson. He grew up in El Paso, Texas, and later in Los Angeles, and graduated high school in Tucson, Arizona. Early on, he boxed professionally to earn money to study art and architecture under Frank Lloyd Wright at the designer's Arizona home. Wright encouraged him to become an actor.

Quinn won two Academy Awards as Best Supporting Actor for the 1952 *Viva Zapata!* and 1956 *Lust for Life*. He was nominated for Best Actor twice and was presented with the Golden Globe Cecil B. DeMille Lifetime Achievement Award. He married the adopted daughter of Cecil B. DeMille, Katherine DeMille, from 1947 to 1965. They had five children, the first of which drowned as a toddler in the next-door comedian W. C. Fields' swimming pool.

Anthony and Katherine divorced when he had an affair with Italian costume designer Jolanda Addolori whom he married in 1966 to 1997. He then married his secretary, Katherine Benvin, in 1997 and they remained married until his death.

This remarkable actor danced in many movies and scenes feature his dancing with Alan Bates in *Zorba the*

Greek. His breakthrough role occurred in 1941 *Blood and Sand* where he played with Tyrone Power and Rita Hayworth. He danced with Rita where he appeared to be a bullfighter dancing around her.

Quotations from Quinn in 1964 *Zorba the Greek:*

Zorba: All right, we go outside where God can see us better.
Zorba: Am I not a man? And is a man not stupid? I'm a man, so I married. Wife, children, house, everything. The full catastrophe.
Quinn: Damn it, boss, I like you too much not to say it. You've got everything except one thing: madness! A man needs a little madness, or else...
Bates: Or else?
Quinn: ...he never dares cut the rope and be free.

Anthony Quinn was one of many Hollywood stars who saw Max Jacobson, M.D. He commented that these vitamin shots gave him "high octane dreams." After he received drugs from him for a while, he wound up calling him "underhanded" and an "evil man" in his 1997 autobiography *One Man Tango*.[2] Quinn decided to disregard De Mille's request to use his injections for good reason. He wanted to be in charge of himself just as his Zorba character wanted.

Quinn played character roles in movies such as 1936 *The Plainsman,* 1941 *They Died with Their Boots* On, 1942 *Road to Morocco, and* 1962 *Lawrence of Arabia.*

He became a naturalized citizen in 1947. In the 1950s, he traveled to Rome where he starred in 1954 *Ulysses,* 1954 *Atilla,* 1954 *La Strada,* and 1956 *The Hunchback of Notre Dame.* He played the role of many foreigners such as Mexicans, Italians, Arabs, Greeks, and more. He played Greeks several times in movies such as *Zorba the Greek* and *The Greek Tycoon,* the latter movie being about the marriage between Aristotle Onassis and Jacqueline Kennedy. He experienced discrimination in Los Angeles and funded various organizations to rally support for equal employment and supported labor activist Cesar Chavez.

He became interested in art and did prize-winning paintings while working with Frank Lloyd Wright. His work was shown in public and private collections. He recorded other songs he sang as well.

Quinn wrote two autobiographies: 1972 *The Original Sin: A Self-Portrait* and *One Man Tango* in 1997. He even wrote scripts and unpublished stories. He died of respiratory failure following radiation treatment for lung cancer.

Notes

1. https://www.nytimes.com/2001/06/04/movies/anthony-quinn-dies-at-86-played -earthy-tough-guys.html)
2. https://www.medicalbag.com/home/features/despicable-doctors/the-secre-service-gave-him-the-code-name-dr-feelgood/)

Edward G. Robinson

Edward G. Robinson (1893-1973) was born Emanuel Goldenberg in Bucharest, Romania, to Jews who came to American when he was ten years old after one of his brothers was attacked by an antisemitic gang. He planned to become a criminal attorney but won an American Academy of Dramatic Arts scholarship, after which he changed his name. He served in the U.S. Navy during WWI but was not sent overseas.

He first worked on stage but with the arrival of sound films, began to make movies playing snarling gangsters. By 1931, his role as Rico in *Little Caesar* made him a star. He occasionally starred in comedies such as 1938 *A Slight Case of Murder* and with Humphrey Bogart, 1938 *The Amazing Dr. Clitterhouse,* and 1959 *A Hole in the Head* with Frank Sinatra. He played an FBI agent in the first American film to portray Nazism as a threat to the United State in 1939 *Confessions of a Nazi Spy*. Here is a movie quotation from 1939 *Confessions of a Nazi Spy:*

> Robinson: I told you I thought this man is an amateur. If he is, why did he become a spy? Well, because he's been listening to speeches, and reading pamphlets about Nazi Germany and believing them. Unfortunately, there are thousands like him in America. Half-witted, hysterical crackpots who go "Hitler-happy" from overindulgence in propaganda that makes them believe that they're supermen.

Here are quotations from 1955 *A Bullet for Joey* when Robinson as an Inspector is talking to actor George Dolenz who played a doctor.

Robinson: I was thinking of Miss Geary. I met her at the golf club yesterday. Do you remember?
Dolenz: Yes.
Robinson: Charming.
Dolenz: Yes, she is.
Robinson: What do you know about her?
Dolenz: Very little, and the little I know, I like.
Robinson: I can't say I blame you. Women make it a pleasure to be a man.

He volunteered for military service at the outset of WWII but was disqualified due to his age of forty-eight. However, he became an active and vocal critic of fascism and Nazism during that era. He donated $100,000 to the USO during WWII and pitched in at the Hollywood Canteen. Being multilingual and speaking seven languages, he worked on broadcasts to countries occupied by the Nazis.

He did crime, war, and poignant films under many directors. However, in 1949, he was investigated by the California Senate's FactFinding Committee on Un-American Activities. They alleged that Robinson was "frequently involved in Communist fronts and causes."

Robinson's career was destroyed by Senator Joseph McCarthy's Commission, despite any proof that he was a member of the Communist party. It took five years for him to clear his name as he struggled to find steady work in Hollywood again. Life won't permit you to live by intellect and by reason alone. Whatever it is, life is not reasonable. Robinson was forced to return to work on the stage, which he had done in the first fifteen years of his life.

Since the Soviet Union was a major U. S. ally in the war against Nazi Germany, many of the more than eight hundred groups he supported and donated to were left-wing groups, some of which were close to the Communist Party. He thought he was helping U.S. allies. He was urged to confess, which essentially meant he was to name the names of those he thought were Communists.

He "confessed" saying that he was duped by people like Albert Maltz, Dalton Trumbo, John Howard Lawsen, Frank Tuttle, Sidney Buchanan, etc. He drafted an article in the *American Legion Magazine* in October 1952 entitled "How the Reds Made a Sucker Out of Me." Those confessions cost him his job because people did not want to hire him, and his money and art collections dwindled.

He was thrilled to be invited to join Cecile B. DeMille's cast for 1956 *The Ten Commandments* filmed in Egypt and Hollywood. DeMille brought Dr. Max Jacobson along to Egypt so that cast and crew could feel energized to work quickly. Robinson received some of those injections and they pepped up the depressed elderly man so that he performed quite well.

Edward G. Robinson said of Cecile B. DeMille, "He saved my career." He remained grateful to DeMille for the rest of his life. Other actors who were considered for the role he played were Raymond Burr, Fredric March, Raymond Massey, Basil Rathbone, Robert Ryan, George Sanders, and Peter Ustinov. He felt incredibly lucky to have been chosen from that set of talented actors.[1]

Robinson was also grateful to Frank Sinatra for the 1959 *A Hole in the Head* where he was second-billed. Robinson was 22 years older than Sinatra but with birthdays the same day, they celebrated on the set with cakes. Sinatra also brought Frank Capra out of retirement to direct this comedy about brothers and it is a delight. Sinatra even sings his old favorite *High Hopes*. Robinson nearly steals the show with his wise-cracking role as the older brother to Sinatra.

Robinson had married stage actress Gladys Lloyd Cassel in 1927 to 1956 and they had a son. He then married Jane Robinson in 1958. She was an artist and fashion designer and the Robinsons accumulated one of the most significant art collections on the West Coast until much of it had to be sold due to his unemployment.

When Charlton Heston was president of the Screen Actors Guild, he presented Robinson with an award in 1969 "in recognition of his pioneering work in organizing the union, his service during World War II, and his outstanding achievement in fostering the finest ideals of the acting profession." Heston and Robinson became good friends over the years.

At the 45th Academy Awards ceremony, Charlton Heston had a flat tire on the way to the awards, so Clint Eastwood began to present the award for Best Picture. Heston ran in at the last minute to present the award. Edward G. Robinson had died on January 26, 1973, but had learned he would receive an honorary award at that ceremony for his greatness in a cinematic lifetime. His widow received his honorary award and told the audience that Robinson was very grateful in his last days when he learned he was to be honored.

His last movie was with friend Charlton Heston in 1973 *Soylent Green*, and he died 84 days after filming that scene. Heston delivered Robinson's eulogy and pall bearers included Jack Warner, Hal Wallis, Mervyn Leroy, George

Burns, Sam Jaffe, and Frank Sinatra. Robinson never won an Academy Award.

Upon his death, he left an estate valued at $2,500,000 which largely consisted of rare works of art. He was a very cultured man and yet could play criminal characters with aplomb. He was in 1948 *Key Largo* with Humphrey Bogart and Lauren Bacall, and Claire Trevor played his girlfriend. She wanted one drink too many and he made her sing for a drink. She sang "Moanin' Low," a song similar to "My Man" sung by Fannie Brice about a man she loved despite his harsh treatment of her. Trevor plowed through the song with difficulty. When she finished, she got no drink when he said: "You were rotten!" He was villainous to the nth degree in that and many films. But his villains always had an Achilles' heel. In this movie, he had a fear of storms which became his undoing.

Robinson was writing his memoir, *All My Yesterday: An Autobiography*, when he died. It was published in 1973 by Hawthorn Books, Inc. It is well-written in a conversational way as if he were chatting with the reader about his life.

Note

1. https://www.jpost.com/judaism/jewish-holidays/article-736448)

Elizabeth Taylor

Elizabeth Taylor (1932-2011) was born in London, England, to a couple from Kansas who moved overseas to open an art gallery in London. Her father was warned by U.S. Ambassador Joseph Kennedy that he should return to the United State due to fear of impending war in Europe, so they moved to Los Angeles in 1939. She was very pretty, and her parents were told that she should be in movies.

She made her acting debut in 1942 with a small role in *There's One Born Every Minute.* The movie was about a couple who advertised falsely that their puddings had a fantastic vitamin that stimulated the female sexual drive. Her next picture, *National Velvet*, with Mickey Rooney, Donald Crisp, and Angela Lansbury was an enormous success. Liz played a horse-loving girl who wins a steeplechase on her specially trained horse. She would go on to play roles with the famous dog Lassie, and later moved to adult roles in movies. She once said, "Some of my best leading men have been dogs and horses."

She would finally win an Academy Award for Best Actress in *Butterfield 8* about a call-girl. Elizabeth starred in that with her fourth husband, Eddie Fisher. She had married hotel millionaire Conrad Hilton Jr. from 1950 to 1951, English actor Michael Wilding 1951-57, and Mike Todd in 1957 who was lost in a plane crash the following year.

Here are some movie quotes. The first is from 1944 *National Velvet:*

I want it all quickly 'cause I don't want God to stop and think and wonder if I'm getting more than my share.

These quotes are from 1954 *The Last Time I Saw Paris* with Van Johnson.

Johnson: You're a girl after my own heart.

Taylor: Make no mistake, I'm after it.

These quotes are from 1960 *Butterfield 8* with Laurence Harvey.

Taylor: You act like a man who's expecting his wife back in town.

Harvey: Look, Gloria, I have to spend at least tonight with her.

Taylor: A good night's sleep will be the best thing for you.

Elizabeth was consoled in her loss after Mike Todd's plane crash by singer Eddie Fisher, who she married from 1959 to 1964. During that marriage, Fisher was constantly supplied with amphetamines and vitamins by Dr. Max Jacobson. She used Jacobson's drugs as well as other drugs, and they both drank much alcohol.

She went to England to make the movie *Cleopatra* with English actor Richard Burton. They fell in love, and she divorced Fisher to marry Richard Burton from 1964 to 1974, and again from 1975 to 1976. The Welshman was an extreme alcoholic, and their marriage was ridden with problems. She had scoliosis, a broken back from her movie *National Velvet*, and used pain killers indiscriminately in addition to alcohol. She finally left Burton and married Senator John Warner from 1976 to 1982, during which she gained a considerable amount of weight, and claimed she led a "boring" life.

She was in and out of the movies to some extent, but finally went to the Betty Ford Hospital for alcohol and drug rehabilitation. In 1992, she married Larry Fortensky, a patient she met there. Their marriage lasted from 1992 to 1996, when he began to drink and do drugs again. After that divorce, she lived a more sedate life with growing heart problems and died of congestive heart failure at the age of 79. She once shocked a son by Michael Wilding when she asked him to inject her with an opiate pain killer. He declined and she administered the needle herself.

The feisty actress was well-known for defending homosexual actors and those who suffered from AIDS so that they might be helped with their problems.

Kay Thompson

Kay Thompson was born Catherine Louise Fink (1909-1998) to a Jewish Austrian pawnbroker and jeweler and his wife, a gentile. She began as a singer on the radio and was a regular on the Bing Crosby-Woodbury Show and the Fred Waring Show. She co-founded *The Lucky Strike Hit Parade* in 1935 with conductor Lennie Hayton. There she met trombonist Jack Jenney whom she married in 1937 and divorced in 1939. In 1937, she and her choir performed songs in the 1937 movie *Manhattan Merry-Go-Round*.

She teamed up with Andre Kostelanetz and his orchestra for *Tune-Up Time,* a radio show produced by radio legend William Spier whom she married in 1942 and divorced in 1947. In 1939, that show had 16-year-old Judy Garland as a guest. They became great friends until Judy died. She became Judy's vocal coach and put the "sob" in Judy's voice, as well as showing her how to sing a song and make it a hit.

Sam Irvin's book *Kay Thompson: From Funny Face to Eloise* described how she was Frank Sinatra's vocal guru, Liza Minnelli's godmother, Noel Coward's playmate, Gene Kelly's charades partner, Fred Astaire's nemesis, Lena Horne's matchmaker, and Andy William's much older girlfriend.[1]

MGM hired Thompson in 1943 as their top vocal arranger, vocal coach, and choral director. Some of her movie arrangements can be seen in 1945 *Ziegfeld Follies,* 1946 *The Harvey Girls,* 1946 *Till the Clouds Roll By,* 1947 *Good News* and 1948 *The Pirate*.

After *The Pirate,* she created a night club act called Kay Thompson and the Williams Brothers. Those four brothers including Andy Williams became an overnight sensation in Las Vegas in 1947, because they did songs that included choreography. Thompson wrote many of their songs and directed them. Their act appeared on stage in many countries as well. She became the coach and Andy's lover (despite being 18 years older). Walter Winchell talked up their act, and the publicity made them the best paid nightclub act up to that time.

Kay Thompson played fashion editor Maggie Prescott in the 1957 musical *Funny Face* with Fred Astaire, Audrey Hepburn, and Gershwin songs, opening the movie with her splashy number "Think Pink!" She was also in the 1970 *Tell Me That You Love Me, Junie Moon* with Liza Minnelli.

Quotations from 1957 *Funny Face:*

> Thompson: Lettie, take an editorial! "To the women of American... No, make it to the women everything. Banish the black, burn the blue, and bury the beige. From now on, girls, think pink!"
> Astaire: We want to sit at your feet and learn. We have so much to learn.
> Thompson: We sit at your feet, humble and ignorant but so willing.
> Hepburn: Look, you two, just leave his feet alone.

Kay lived in the Plaza Hotel and created a book in 1955 called *Kay Thompson's Eloise: A Book for Precocious Grown-Ups* which became a sensation. It was quickly followed by the 1957 *Eloise in Paris*, 1958 *Eloise at Christmastime*, and 1959 *Eloise in Moscow*. She collaborated with Hilary Knight for the cartoons of Eloise. Mischievous little Eloise was a six-year-old with spiky hair and a pot-belly who loved pink and roamed around the rooms of the Plaza Hotel meeting and commenting about hotel guests.[2]

The Plaza Hotel was so delighted to have a book about the little imp that she was given a free room for nearly twenty years. Having been the godmother of Liza Minnelli, both women were close and used Dr. Max Jacobson's vitamin injections that produced addictions. When Kay became unable to produce any more Eloise adventures and became terribly emaciated and unproductive, the hotel no longer offered her free housing in 1973.

Thanks to Liza Minnelli, Kay lived the rest of her life with Liza rent-free until her death in 1998. People only learned of her personal relationship with Andy Williams through his 2009 autobiography entitled *Moon River and Me*. Their relationship ceased when Andy met and married French-American singer Claudine Longet in 1961 until their divorce in 1975.

In the 1970s, Plaza Hotel visitors often stopped by the Eloise ice cream parlor off Palm Court. Room 934 was displayed as Eloise's room.[3]

Notes

1. "Kay Thompson: From Funny Face to Eloise" by Sam Irvin reviewed by Joanne Latimer, by Maclean's January 13, 2011)
2. https://www.tabletmag.com/sections/community/articles/the-woman-behind-eloise
3. https://web.archive.org/20060910012957/

Billy Wilder

Billy Wilder was born Samuel Wilder (1906-2002) in what is now Poland near Vienna, Austria, to Polish Jews who owned a chain of railroad cafes. His father also managed a hotel before they moved to Vienna. In 1924, Billy became a journalist beginning in the crossword puzzle department and working his way into movie reviews and entertainment.

In 1926, jazz band leader Paul Whiteman was on tour in Vienna and Wilder interviewed him. Billy became a fan of the Whiteman band. Whiteman liked him and took him with the band to Berlin. He earned a living as a taxi dancer in Berlin where hotel ballrooms directors sent dancers to the tables of ladies who paid to dance.[1]

In 1927, he worked tea dances in the roof garden of the Eden Hotel near the Zoo. It was built in 1912 and the roof garden also feared miniature golf. The hotel bar was considered one of the most elegant bars in town, and the prices were accordingly high. Successful writers, actors, and artists such as Erich Maria Remarque, Marlene Dietrich, and Peter Lorre were customers.[2]

Now, a new book has been published called *Billy Wilder on Assignment: Dispatches from Weimar Berlin and Interwar Vienna*. Drawing on his own experiences, Wilder wrote a story about his work in this anthology called "Waiter, A Dancer, Please." The story began thusly:

> Herr Isin's red eyes gaze at me as though straining to say: Go!

Yes, yes, I'll go dance. Over there in the corner, the lady in the Persian lamb coat and the crocodile leather shoes. I'll go ask her to dance.

But Herr Isin taps my shoulder. "You're dancing with table 91. Right over here..."[3]

Soon, those taxi dancing days were over. By 1929, he was working as a screenwriter and produced twelve German movies by 1933. However, as Adolf Hitler rose to power, Wilder moved on to Paris but knew Max Jacobson in Germany and wrote this about the doctor:

I knew him extremely well—in Berlin, he was my doctor. Talk about writers in exile! Here's this doctor in exile, he cannot get a diploma so he performs abortions. You know how old this guy is today? He has to be in the early 70s! But what a difference from his days in Paris, eh? Whenever he comes out here to L.A. I see him. Or I meet him on planes. He is accompanying Mr. Cecil B. DeMille to Egypt because Mr. DeMille is going to do a new version of *The Ten Commandments,* during which Mr. DeMille has himself a heart attack, but Dr. Feelgood pumps him full of amphetamine magic shots, so Mr. DeMille can still climb ladders and shoot the scenes, with maybe 6,000 extras all standing around.

Wilder moved from Paris where he directed movies until he landed in Hollywood in 1934. His parents and other family members died in the Holocaust. He has an excellent reputation and most people who have seen his work would agree that his movies are never boring.

When he arrived in the U.S., he was permitted a six-month stay. When that ran out, he moved to Mexico to await further papers to live in the United States. He included this in his 1941 movie called *Hold Back the Dawn*. That movie has a U.S. teacher played by Olivia de Havilland swept off her feet by a gigolo played by Charles Boyer in a Mexican border town. Unaware that he is looking for a woman who will help him get a green card, she marries him after only a few days. While carrying out the charade, he begins to fall for her, angering his girlfriend, played by Paulette Goddard. As his plan is foiled, he realized that keeping his wife may be more important than his green card.

When Wilder returned to the U.S. from Mexico, his first success was *Ninotchka* with Greta Garbo in a romantic comedy he did with German immigrant Ernst Lubitsch. It was advertised saying "Garbo laughs." It was later remade as the musical *Silk Stockings* with Fred Astaire and Cyd Charisse. Wilder went on to film 1942 *Ball of Fire*, 1942 *The Major and the Minor* and 1944 *Double Indemnity*. The latter movie with Fred MacMurray, Barbara Stanwick, and Edward G. Robinson was a major hit. He co-wrote it with mystery writer Raymond Chandler based on James M. Cain's novel.

In 1945, the Psychological Warfare Department of the U.S. Department of War produced a documentary directed by Wilder. It was intended to educate German audiences about Nazi atrocities. Two years later he directed Ray Milland in *The Lost Weekend* about an alcoholic which received four Academy Award including Best Picture.[5]

In 1950, Wilder co-wrote and directed *Sunset Boulevard* bringing back silent film actress Gloria Swanson and silent movie director Erich von Stroheim together with William Holden who played a gigolo. The movie ended with Swanson's words: "All right, Mr. DeMille, I'm ready for my close-up." Wilder, a writer and director, just had a way with words.

Wilder had other famous movie last lines. In *The Apartment,* Jack Lemmon and Shirley MacLaine finally wind up together in his apartment which was often used by Lemmon's supervisor, Fred MacMurray for adulterous trysts. Lemmon's co-worker, MacLaine, learned that Lemmon would no longer allow MacMurray to bring her to his apartment for a quickie. MacLaine ran from MacMurray to Lemmon, to his apartment where they happily began to play cards together. Lemmon said, "I absolutely adore you." MacLaine said, "Shut up and deal."

Perhaps the funniest closing line in a movie was from his 1959 *Some Like It Hot*. The final scene showed Jack Lemmon telling Joe E. Brown that he is a man. Brown fell for Lemmon who dressed like a woman to avoid gangsters. Brown simply smiled and said, "Well, nobody's perfect." That line was used in the French newspaper *Le Monde* in Wilder's obituary which was entitled "Billy Wilder is dead. Nobody's perfect."

Notes

1. https://davidhayes.ca/2022/03/waiter-a-dancer-please/
2. http://www.weimarberlin.com/2021/03/hotel-eden.html
3. https://davidhayes.ca/2022/03/waiter-a-dancer-please/
4. https://playingintheworldgame.com/tag/max-jacobson/
5. https://www.bookforum.com/print/2901/how-billy-wilder-survived-the-twentieth-century/

Tennessee Williams

Thomas Lanier Williams III (1911-1983) took the pen name of Tennessee Williams. He was a relative of poet Sidney Lanier, for whom he was named. His father was an alcoholic traveling shoe salesman married to the daughter of an Episcopal priest. There existed a struggle between good and bad in his household and his mind.

Williams suffered from diphtheria as a child and became very frail. His father lost jobs and they moved many times, wherein he was often beaten and criticized as effeminate by his father.

He went to college and entered his poetry and stories in contests to win money. He finally moved to New Orleans where he wrote for the Works Progress Administration begun by President Roosevelt. He continued writing while attending universities to graduate with a bachelor's degree but could not make a living. His father put him to work in a shoe factory. After a nervous breakdown at age 24, he became extremely lonely and began to have love affairs with men.

By 1944, he began to find success when New York City director Elia Kazan staged *The Glass Menagerie* on Broadway. That was followed by *A Streetcar Named Desire* in 1947. More of his plays ran on Broadway and movies were made of some including *Summer and Smoke, The Rose Tattoo, Cat on a Hot Tin Roof, Sweet Bird of Youth,* etc. These early works poured out of the lonely man, but he wrote them slowly and methodically as was his way.

He began to write more, drink more, and used drugs administered by Dr. Max Jacobson to fight off depression. Tennessee described his first injection thusly: "I felt as if a concrete sarcophagus about me had sprung open and I was released as a bird on the wing."[1]

He learned to inject himself and Jacobson sent him needles and ampules to take. Tennessee wrote to his editor at New Directions saying that he hoped to get through his final Broadway production of *The Night of the Iguana,* and thought he needed someone like Dr. Max Jacobson to make it. Jacobson had warned him not to combine the injections with alcohol, but he often did so. He began to get rather mixed up and emotional, so he was given an anti-psychotic medicine called Mellaril by some physician. Williams referred to this high-low drug combination as the "Goforth Syndrome."

Williams fell in love with actor Frank Merlo, who became his agent until Merlo developed lung cancer. After their relationship of fifteen years, Merlo died in 1963. Tennessee nursed Merlo through the illness and was very forlorn when his lover died. Consumed by depression, he not only used drugs and alcohol, but went into psychoanalysis with famous analyst Dr. Lawrence Kubie.[2] He thought of himself as a sinner and Kubie tried to reverse that by helping him learn to control his urges for instant relief through drugs.

He ceased treatment with Kubie after a year. Kubie tried to show him that self-knowledge must go on throughout one's entire life. He was unclear in *The Night of the Iguana* as well, so that his characters each wrestled with their conscience about how to behave. Fighting their own inner demons was quite different than his other books where characters wrestled with each other.

Williams found a new relationship with another man after Merlo but there were infidelities and drug use on both sides. He felt he learned things in analysis but grew inconsolable. His beloved sister Rose was diagnosed with schizophrenia and was later lobotomized. He cared for her, visiting her frequently and paying for her institutional treatment until he died.

He continued to be lonely as an aging gay man, and there were many men for one-night stands. He continued using Dr. Jacobson's amphetamine-laced injections and took Seconal tablets for insomnia. He lived in the New York City Hotel Elysee where he died by choking on a plastic cap for his barbiturates container which got caught in his throat. He was found dead with a toxic level of Seconal in his body.[3]

Williams left instructions for his body to be placed in a canvas sack and dropped overboard where poet and author Hart Crane (1899-1932) had died by suicide in the Gulf of Mexico. Crane was a gay poet whom Tennessee admired. His instructions were followed after his demise.

Notes

1. *Tennessee Williams: Mad Pilgrimage of the Flesh,* by John Lahr, W. W. Norton & Co., 2014.
2. "Incorporating Brain Explanations in Psychoanalysis: Tennessee Williams as a Case Study" by W. Scott Griffies. *Psychodyn. Psychiatry*, 2022 Fall;50(3):492-512. Doi: 10.1521/prps.2022.50.3.492. htttpes://pubmed.ncbi.nlm.nih.gov/36047801/
3. https://archive.nytimes.com/www.nytimes.com/books/00/12/31/specials/williams-drugs.html

CHAPTER SIX
Timothy Leary, Ph.D. and Mortimer Hartman, M.D.

Timothy Leary (1920-1996) received a Ph.D. in psychology from the University of California and went on to lecture at Harvard in 1959. His early research in personality and social relationships included work as a psychotherapist. There, he met Richard Alpert who also had a PhD. in psychology from Stanford University and came to Harvard in 1953 as an assistant professor and they joined forces to study personality.

They began the Harvard Psilocybin Project to study a hallucinogen which occurs in a certain species of mushrooms. They tried to understand its effect upon human consciousness with volunteer subjects by recording their descriptions of the experience. At that time, psilocybin and lysergic diethylamide acid (LSD) were legal substances manufactured by Sandoz Laboratories.

As the two Harvard men studied these effects, they also used hallucinogens and recorded their own experiences. Gradually, their research was criticized for using unorthodox methods. Editorials in the *Harvard Crimson* accused Alpert and Leary of promoting the recreational use of these substances. In the spring of 1963, Alpert and Leary were fired for lack of scientific rigor and failure to follow research guidelines. Leary was an outspoken critic of most forms of social control and criticized his critics.[1]

Leary was arrested for marijuana possession and declared the Marijuana Tax Act was unconstitutional. On May 19, 1969, the Supreme Court agreed with Leary vs. United States and his 1965 conviction was seemingly quashed. That day, he announced that he would run against Ronald Reagan for Governor of California. His campaign slogan was "Come together, join the party."

Leary later received a ten-year sentence for possession of marijuana and another ten was added for the previous arrest making twenty years to be served consecutively. Leary, based on psychological tests where he showed interest in gardening, was assigned to work as a gardener in a lower security prison, from which he escaped in September 1970.[2]

Leary was vigorously pursued by law enforcement officers. He was arrested by Gordon Liddy, a sheriff's deputy and later of Watergate fame, for drugs and imprisoned. In a dramatic escape from prison, he was helped to join Eldredge Cleaver in Algeria where he experienced the American government-in-exile along with Black Panthers. Unhappy with them, he fled to Switzerland, then to Afghanistan, and was captured there and returned to the United States in 1973. He was a prison mate of Charles Manson until release by California Governor Edmund G. Brown, Jr. in 1976.[3]

He continued to experiment with LSD and had many followers such as actress Susan Sarandon and actor Dan Aykroyd. His motto was "turn on, tune in, drop out."

Toward the end of his life, he became involved with cybernetics, which he thought was the new way to expand consciousness. He played with virtual reality, designed computer games, and criticized the Nancy Reagan era proposal for children tempted by drugs to "Just say no." He proposed that people "Just say know."

Leary's sad life included a first wife who committed suicide, two marriages and divorces, a daughter's suicide in 1990, and he was separated from his fourth wife when he learned he had inoperable prostate cancer. He made plans for a public death with tapings of visitors, drug intake, readings, and meditations.

Other scientists were experimenting with LSD such as Dr. Mortimer Hartman who ran the Psychiatric Institute of Beverly Hills. He had undergone psychoanalysis himself, and felt he understood the mind-opening possibilities of LSD in addition to therapy.

Actress Betsy Drake was interested in psychoanalysis and mind exploration. She took LSD under supervision in Dr. Hartman's office. This was in response to realization that her husband, Cary Grant, was having an affair with Sophia Loren while filming a movie in Spain. When he returned, she told him of the valuable experience she had with LSD, and he went to Dr. Hartman as many as 100 times for LSD sessions.[4]

He talked freely about the excellent experiences and realizations he had under the influence of that psychedelic. Actress swimming star Esther Williams contacted her friend, Cary Grant, to ask for a reference to his doctor. She then went to see Dr. Hartman and under the influence of that drug in his office, learned much about herself that was immensely helpful.

In the early 1960s, the Food and Drug Administration started to investigate the Psychiatric Institute of Beverly Hills, forcing Dr. Hartman to close it in 1962. By 1966, the drug was illegal. By then, Hartman had left California.

Cary Grant continued to take LSD from other sources and left $10,000 to Hartman in his will, describing the doctor as his "wise mahatma."

There are many people who believe that LSD can open doors to self-understanding. Among LSD users who have described their experiences are computer experts Bill Gates and Steve Jobs, Tesla CEO Elon Musk, Francis Crick who discovered the structure of DNA, Ambassador and author Clare Booth Luce, actress Carrie Fisher, Aldous Huxley, Andre Previn, James Coburn, Anais Nin, Ken Kesey, and some of the Beatles musical group.[5]

Sandoz is a pharmaceutical company based in Basel, Switzerland, the site of LSD's discovery in 1938. In 1929, Sandoz hired Albert Hofmann. He and other Sandoz researchers identified lysergic acid as the common chemical basis among all the biologically active ergot compounds. In 1938, Hofmann synthesized LSD-25 among other ergot compounds and analogs from lysergic acid.

Five years later on April 16, 1943, Hofmann accidentally discovered LSD's psychedelic effects while experimenting in the Sandoz laboratory. Days later, he took a dose himself, and described his experiences in his book *LSD—My Problem Child*. Sandoz began clinical trials on the substance at the University Psychiatric Clinic in Zurich in 1947.

During World War II, Sandoz launched large-scale production of LSD. It was called "Delysid" and was used to induce psychoses and treat schizophrenia. A 1964 catalog of Sandoz described its use "in analytical psychotherapy to elicit release of repressed material and to provide mental relaxation, particularly in anxiety states and obsessional neuroses."

It was taken off the market in 1965 after LSD had escaped the labs and fueled the counterculture fad of the 1960s. There were some 10,000 publications on the substance by 1970. The Sandoz website does not mention its history with psychedelic pharmaceuticals. During the LSD era, it was shocking to learn how many in the movie business were using this drug.[6]

Notes

1. https://www.wired.com/2013/10/timothey-leary-archives)
2. lifeofthebeatles.blogspot.com/2009/08/beatle-people-timothy-leary.html
3. https://www.nytimes.cojm/1996/06/01/us/timothey-learny-pied-piper-of-psychedelic-60-s-dies-at-75.html?sec=&spon=&pagewanted=all
4. https://www.vice.comj/en/article/vdpqpj/cary-grant-lsd-old-hollywood-289.
5. psychedelicpassage.com/21-surprising-people-who-have-taken-psychedelics/
6. https://jezebel.com/everyone-in-old-hollywood-was-on-0acid-5582694

Dan Aykroyd

Daniel Aykroyd was born in 1952 in Ottawa, Canada, to a civil engineer and policy advisor to Canadian Prime Minister Pierre Trudeau and a secretary. Dan used to watch his father directing blasts through granite rock to run highways along the Gatineau Parkway.

His great grandfather was a dentist and a mystic who corresponded with author Sir Arthur Conan Doyle on Spiritualism. Doyle was a physician who authored stories about detective Sherlock Holmes and friend, Dr. Watson. Dentists in those days used hypnosis with patients to decrease their pain so they had some knowledge of mesmerism and people in altered states of consciousness.

Dan's father was exploring his grandfather's basement to decide what should be saved when he found his grandfather's hand-written descriptions of seances and mediums, where attempts to communicate with the dead were carried out. Aykroyd grew up in a household where these subjects were discussed. It formed his ideas for skits and the *Ghostbuster* movies which were big hits in 1984, 1989, 2016, and 2023.

Dan wrote the foreword for his father's 2009 book entitled *A History of Ghosts: The True Story of Seances, Mediums, Ghosts, and Ghostbusters*. Dan not only considers himself a spiritualist, but believes that communication with the dead can occur, and thinks earth has been visited by extraterrestrials over the centuries.

Dan Aykroyd became a writer and jokester on the late-night comedy show *Saturday Night Live*. He did excellent impersonations of celebrities and attended certain clubs in Ottawa that featured blues artists. He met comedian John

Belushi with similar tastes and they hung out together. The two men worked with a band popularized in the 1980 movie *The Blues Brothers,* which Aykroyd co-wrote, followed by a sequel. They also established a House of Blues chain of music venues and the Crystal Head Vodka brand.

Both men used drugs, but John Belushi used less caution and died of an overdose. Dan Aykroyd was interested in LSD and joined other Hollywood stars like Susan Sarandon in exploring the use of that drug with Timothy Leary. Dan's wife, Donna Dixon, whom he married in 1983, often joined him early on in these outings. They separated in 2022 and have three children.

When Timothy Leary died, he asked others to film him with his friends, showing his use of drugs, and capturing his final words and his lethal dose of LSD. A celebration of his death was held by his followers and users.

Johnny Depp

John Christopher Depp II was born in 1963 to a civil engineer and waitress. His parents divorced when he was fifteen, and his mother later married a man whom Depp called "an inspiration." Johnny dropped out of high school to become a rock musician. He played in a band and through his wife met actor Nicolas Cage, who encouraged him to pursue acting. Although he did not plan to be an actor, he wanted to earn money to cover his musical training and career.

After a few small parts in movies, he became a teen idol in a TV series called *21 Jump Street,* playing a police officer. He made interesting choices about movie roles and played in Tim Burton's 1990 *Edward Scissorhands* with Winona Ryder. He watched Charlie Chaplin films to learn how to create sympathy without dialogue. After some parts in horror films, he starred with Leonardo DiCaprio in the 1993 *What's Eating Gilbert Grape*. He returned to Tim Burton to play the title role in the 1994 *Ed Wood*, about a very inept film director. He starred with Al Pacino in the 1997 *Donnie Brasco*.

Continuing to learn by watching stars like Angela Lansbury, Roddy McDowall, and Basil Rathbone, he fashioned unusual performances in 2000 *The Man Who Cried,* 2000 *Chocolat,* and 2001 *Blow*. In 2001 *From Hell*, he played an inspector who investigated Jack the Ripper murders in London. He starred in the Walt Disney 2003 *Pirates of the Caribbean: The Curse of the Black Pearl*. He played the role of Scottish author J. M. Barrie in the 2004 *Finding Neverland* and appeared in the French film 2004 *Happily Ever After*. He then founded his own film production company under Warner Brothers Pictures.

He worked again with Tim Burton for the musical in 2007 *Sweeney Todd: The Demon Barber of Fleet Street* where he used a vocal coach to sing. He was inspired by Peter Lorre's creepy role in the 1935 *Mad Love*. He has continued to portray unusual main characters such that he is commended by critics and has been the highest paid actor ever in movies. This is despite setbacks from movies that were panned and his abuse of alcohol and drugs which have interfered with his personal life and his career.

He married Lori Allison from 1983 to 1985, Amber Heard from 2015 to 2017, and had partners with well-known ladies since then.

He has co-owned a Los Angeles nightclub, Man Ray restaurant in Paris, and edited folk singer Woody Guthrie's novel *House of Earth* published in 2013. He has written songs, played guitar, done the soundtrack of some films, and is a member of several musical groups. He played at the Royal Albert Hall in London in 2023 along with Eric Clapton, Rod Stewart, Ronnie Wood, and Kirk Hammett.

He created some artwork that sold out in one day at the Castle Fine Art gallery in London's Covent Garden. Those works included paintings of people who inspired him such as Al Pacino, Elizabeth Taylor, Boy Dylan, and Keith Richards.

His achievements put him in the category of a genius, but his substance abuse, injurious behavior, recklessness, and lawsuits have cost money and brought criticism. He admitted his addictions to opiates, misuse of alcohol, and use of marijuana, MDMA (Ecstasy), LSD, and cocaine. On July 18, 2023, he was unable to perform in Budapest, Hungary, when he was found unconscious in his hotel room. He was on a planned European tour with a musical group called the Hollywood Vampires. It is hoped that this remarkable and perceptive man can recover his life effectively.[1,2] There is news that he is again performing.

There is a 12-minute movie called *Stuff* directed by Johnny Depp and Gibby Haynes in 1993. It was about a house near Depp's residence where John Frusciante lived, and people did drugs there in private. Cameras drifted through the house as a weird soundtrack played, picturing messed up furniture, holes in walls, graffiti on walls, and debris everywhere. The final scene shows Timothy Leary sitting on a desk while Frusciante lies on a couch. Was that meant to resemble how a psychoanalyst and a patient lying on a couch might have worked? This party place had become so bad that even hard-core junkies might have run away from this house.[3]

Notes

1. https://www.marca.com/en/lifestyle/celebrities/2023/07/26/64c0e2f746163fa7088b456d.html
2. https://www.hellomagazine.com/celebrities/498085/johnny-depp-shares-sudden-news-fans-left-concerned-hollywood-vampires/
3. https://dangerousminds.net/comments/john_frusciante_meets_timothy_leary_in_johnny_depp_and_gibby_haynes_stuff

Betsy Drake

Betsy Drake (1923-2015) was an American actress, writer, and psychotherapist. She was the third wife of actor Cary Grant in his longest marriage from 1949 to 1962. Her parents were American expatriates living in Paris when she was born. Her grandfather and his brother had opened the Drake Hotel in Chicago in 1920. They lost their money in the 1929 stock-market crash and her family returned to the U.S.

She went to many schools including National Park Seminary, and gradually chose to focus on acting. She was selected by Elia Kazan as one of the founding members of Actors Studio. Cary Grant saw her on the stage in London in 1947 on a trip he made to visit his mother. Grant and Drake both happened to sail on the *Queen Mary* back to the U.S. and he helped her arrange a contract with RKO and David Selznick.[1]

Grant co-starred with Drake in her first movie, *Every Girl Should Be Married* (1948), also starring Franchot Tone and Alan Mowbray.

Grant and Drake fell in love and wanted to marry. Howard Hughes, a very close friend of Grant, flew them to Phoenix, Arizona, on Christmas Day in 1949, for a private ceremony where he served as best man for the groom.[2]

Hughes had flown his B-23 plane in 1946 with Cary Grant to pick up Mrs. David Selznick at the Orange Municipal Airport. They had flown about in Boston to several sites for a movie Grant was going to make. In a later flight, Hughes nearly killed himself while testing a new plane over Beverly Hills. He was hospitalized for some time and then convalesced at Cary Grant's home in 1946.

Hughes was making movies and was involved with many female movie stars, one of whom, Jean Peters, he later married.[3]

In 1954, they bought an idyllic Spanish house just east of Palm Springs. Betsy and Cary explored yoga, mysticism, transcendentalism, and other things. He used hypnosis to give up smoking. She co-starred with him in the radio series *Mr. and Mrs. Blandings* in 1951. They appeared together in *Room for One More* (1952) and Drake appeared in the 1957 movie *Will Success Spoil Rock Hunter*.

In *Room for One More*, Grant makes the clever comments while Drake gives him the straight lines in many scenes.

> Drake: What's that supposed to be?
> Grant: A woman.
> Drake: Not a very good likeness...
> Grant: I had to draw it from memory.

In another scene, they are discussing a child.
Drake: This child has been through a lot. She's a disturbed adolescent.
Grant: I'm a disturbed adult.
Drake wrote the script for the 1958 movie *Houseboat* in which she expected to co-star with Grant. However, Grant had begun an affair with the thirty years younger Sophia Loren while filming *The Pride and the Passion* and arranged for Loren to replace Drake in the *Houseboat* movie. Unaware of this, Drake flew to Spain during the filming of *The Pride and the Passion*. While there, she realized that her husband was in love with Sophia.[4]

She sailed back to the U.S. on the infamous Italian liner *SS Andrea Doria*. When the *Doria* collided with the *Stockholm,* she was among more than seven hundred terrified people rescued by the French liner *Ile de France.* She returned home and was severely distressed about the collapse of her marriage as well as having had a post-traumatic stress reaction from her narrow escape with death.

In Drake's frustration, she sought help at the Psychiatric Institute of Dr. Mortimer Hartman. The doctor recommended LSD and she explored the depressing events of her recent life. Grant returned home after the affair ended. Loren had declined Grant's marriage proposal in favor of Italian movie producer Carlo Ponti.

Drake found her treatment so helpful that she after several months of LSD therapy she said, "LSD therapy gave me the courage to leave my husband and speak my mind to him."[5]

Cary saw the changes in Betsy and also wondered in a paranoid sort of way how she talked about him to the doctor. So, he made an appointment and began LSD treatments. He had a breakthrough of emotions unlike anything he had ever experienced. He spoke highly of it to friends and others in the media.

Betsy and Cary separated in 1958, remained friends, and divorced in 1962. She decided to retire from movies and studied at Harvard earning an M.Ed. She became a psychotherapist for children and taught at UCLA and Pepperdine University. She did not remarry but used her acting experience in psychodrama. She wrote an article in March 1975 in the *American Journal of Orthopsychiatry* entitled "Psychoanalytically Oriented Psychodrama with Multiple Family Groups."

She worked to help homeless children in Los Angeles, and wrote a novel, *Children, You Are Very Little* in

1971 published by Atheneum Books. She was also in the documentary *Cary Grant: A Class Apart* wherein she described her time with Grant and denied rumors that he was bisexual. She eventually moved to London where she died in 2015.[6]

Notes

1. https://www.atholdailynews.com/Celebrity-visits-to-Orange-Airport-47210332
2. https://www.desertsun.com/story/life/2022/07/03/palm-springs-history-quiet-desert-life-betsy-drake-and-cary-grand/7791166001/
3. https://academic.oup.com/book/33530/chapter-abstract/287878202?redirectedFrom=fulltext https://spartacus-educational.com/JFKhughesH.htm
4. https://theguardian.com/film/2014/oct/19/sophia-or-reveals-the-story-of-cary-grants-passion
5. https://medium.com/picture-palace/cary-grants-lsd-obsession-e2fbf9d5ac68
6. http://www.tcm.com/thismonth/article?cid=76185

Cary Grant

Cary Grant (1904-1986) was born Archibald Leach in Bristol, England. His alcoholic father was a tailor's presser in a clothing factory and his mother was a seamstress. When he was one, his four-year-old brother died of tuberculosis. His mother was severely depressed but occasionally took him to the movies and taught him songs and dances. She disliked alcohol and tobacco and reduced his allowance when he misbehaved.

When he was nine, his father placed his mother in a mental institution but told the boy that she had gone away on "a long holiday." He later told young Archie that she had died. He grew up resenting his mother for having left him. When he was ten, his father got married and started a new family while leaving him with his paternal grandparents. He would not learn that his mother was still alive until he was thirty-one, when his father made a deathbed confession.

Cary Grant visited his mother's institution and arranged for her to leave there in June 1935. He visited her again in October 1938, and supported her until she died.

During his childhood, at age 11, he won a scholarship to a grammar school requiring a uniform which his father could barely afford. He was good at sports and especially fives, which was a sort of handball. He was popular, attractive, acrobatic, and mischievous. He worked backstage in Bristol theaters and at age 13, worked with a magician. Cary went down to Southampton for dock work and tried to become a ship's cabin boy but was too young.

At age 14, he was expelled from school for misdeeds. He joined an acrobatic troupe that began touring the country where he learned pantomime and physical skills.

The group sailed to the U.S. on the *RMS Olympic* when he was sixteen. Douglas Fairbanks and Mary Pickford were aboard the ship, returning from their honeymoon, and Grant played shuffleboard with Fairbanks who became his role model. He later met the Marx brothers, enjoyed their comedy style, and thought quite well of the handsome Zeppo Marx.

He began to fashion himself like Douglas and Zeppo, spending money on good clothing, keeping a trim figure, and sunning for a nice tan on face, chest, and limbs. He began to perform in New York in vaudeville, juggling, acrobatics, stilt walking, riding a unicycle, and improving his comic techniques.

He finally landed a movie contract starring in the 1932 *This Is the Night*. Later that year, he starred in *Hot Saturday* with Randolph Scott, the beginning of a lifetime friendship. Scott had gotten into movies because his father, the first CPA in North Carolina, knew Howard Hughes. Howard opened doors for Scott with Cecil B. DeMille and others. Grant and Scott lived together for several years and played in one other movie together—*My Favorite Wife*. Grant also became friends with Howard Hughes.[1]

Cary Grant began to star in movies as a talented comedian who sometimes played serious roles. He first married Virginia Cherrill from 1934 to 1935, and heiress Barbara Hutton from 1942 to 1945. He next married Betsy Drake from 1949 to 1962. His last marriage was to Dyan Cannon from 1965 to 1968. At their divorce proceedings, Dyan stated that he used LSD which caused problems in their relationship. He asked her to use LSD with him to save their marriage and she did. She authored a book, *Dear Cary,* in which she wrote:

I think he thought it (LSD) was a gateway to peace inside himself... He thought it was a gateway to God."²

They had a daughter, Jennifer Grant, who brought him great joy as he recorded her life and special events until he died.

Grant told many about the virtues of LSD. He said that he experienced his own birth again under the influence of LSD. He told *The New York Times Magazine* decades later,

> It was absolute release. You are still able to feed yourself, of course, drive your car, that kind of thing, but you've lost a lot of the tension... We come into this world with nothing on our tape. We are computers, after all. The content of that tape is supplied by our mothers mainly, because our fathers are off hunting or shooting or work. Now the mother can teach only what she knows, and many of these patterns of behavior are not good, but they're still passed on to the child. I came to the conclusion that I had to be reborn, to wipe clean the tape.³

At another point in his life, he explained that he attended Dr. Hartman's office, selecting music to hear while he took his prescribed dose of LSD in a small dark room. He said:

> LSD permits you to fly apart. I got clearer and clearer... I forced myself through the realization that I loved my parents and forgave them for what they didn't know. I became happier for it, and the insights

I gained dispelled many of the fears I had prior to that time.[4]

After years of success in movies, Grant's career began to sag. He took some years off from movies but Alfred Hitchcock, who made a total of four pictures with Grant, revived his career. He co-starred with Grace Kelly in *To Catch a Thief*. His other Hitchcock films were *Suspicion, Notorious,* and the last was *North by Northwest*. Hitchcock said Cary Grant was the only star he really loved.

In 1946 *Notorious,* Grant and Bergman have the longest kiss in movie history. The movie plot is for her to be a spy on Nazis, and authorities like Louis Calhern who sought her for that mission discuss her character in this scene:

Calhern: I don't like this. I don't like her coming here.
Moroni: She's had me worried for some time. A woman of that sort.
Grant: What sort is that?
Moroni: I don't think any of us have any illusions about her character, have we, Devlin?
Grant: Not at all, not in the slightest. Miss Huberman is first, last, and always not a lady. She may be risking her life, but when it comes to being a lady, she doesn't hold a candle to your wife, sitting in Washington, playing bridge with three other ladies of great honor and virtue.

After Grant's divorce from Dyan Cannon, Grant married thirteen years later to Barbara Harris, a British hotel public relations agent some 47 years younger than himself. They travelled to Monaco four times to visit

Princess Grace and Prince Rainier. In fact, during the late 1970s and early 1980s, he suffered the deaths of dear ones such as Howard Hughes, Howard Hawks, Barbara Hutton, Alfred Hitchcock, Grace Kelly, Ingrid Bergman, and David Niven. Grant died of a massive stroke on November 29, 1986, while he was preparing for an evening on stage called *A Conversation with Cary Grant*.

After daughter Jennifer was born, he retired from acting at age 62 in 1966. He then pursued other business interests by representing the cosmetic firm of Fabergé and sitting on the board of Metro-Goldwyn-Mayer. He died at age 82 and his daughter, who finally got into television acting, wrote a book called *Good Stuff: A Reminiscence of My Father, Cary Grant*. In her book, she firmly stated that he was not homosexual and at most, might have had a fling with a man which she hoped he enjoyed. He left his assets to wife Barbara Harris and daughter Jennifer Grant.

Notes

1. https://elisa-rolle.livejournal.com/1812429.html
2. https://www.smh.com.au/entertainment/books/cary-grants-lsd-gateway-to-god-20111018-1lye1.html
3. https://www.vulture.com/2017/06/cary-grants-lsd-therapy-the-inside-story.html
4. https://www.townandcountrymag.com/leisure/arts-and-culture/a38r63704/cary-grant-lsd-flying-over-sunset-broadway/

Susan Sarandon

Susan Sarandon was born Susan Tomalin in 1946 to an advertising executive, television producer, and one-time nightclub singer. She was brought up Roman Catholic, and she and her sister won swimming contests when young. She joined a band in high school and a dance group who entertained sick children. She was in school plays and earned a B.A. in drama at the Catholic University of America in Washington, D.C.

She married Chris Sarandon from 1967 to 1979, and they were both interested in acting. She managed to get bit parts before becoming a star. She won an Academy Award for Best Actress in the 1995 *Dead Man Walking* and was nominated for her roles in 1980 *Atlantic City*, 1991 *Thelma and Louise*, 1992 *Lorenzo's Oil*, and 1994 *The Client*. She has narrated many documentaries and starred in television films.

Her role in 1991 *Thelma and Louise* with Gena Davis is riveting as the movie ends. Police are chasing them as they drive through the desert.

> Davis: Okay, then, listen. Let's not get caught.
> Sarandon: What are you talkin' about?
> Davis: Go!
> Sarandon: You sure?
> Davis: Yeah, yeah. [They hug and kiss, then Sarandon steps on the gas.]

Susan had other partners such as Louis Malle 1977-1980, Franco Amurri 1984-1988, Tim Robbins 1988-2009, and Jonathan Bricklin 2010-2015. She has three children.

She and Bricklin helped establish ping-pong lounges named SPiN.

On the Jimmy Kimmel Live television show, she described her trip to the 2014 Burning Man festival at Black Rock Desert, Nevada. She described being a friend of Timothy Leary and using psychedelic drugs. She took his ashes to a temple that she and some people built at Burning Man. She said they diluted the ashes for a toast at the end of the day, so they drank Leary's ashes.[1]

Many people including Leary's friend Dan Aykroyd participated in the ceremony of a 60-foot-tall man-like structure honoring Leary's time in Mexico. Sarandon led the march wearing a white gown with a crown of roses. His ashes were put into a temporary church built as an art installation in the desert for the week-long festival. The church was to burn as part of the event after the giant "man" was burned in a glowing late-night party. Leary had gifted her with some of his ashes when he died in 1996.[2]

She said, "I think he'd be so happy. I think he would have loved the chaos... and all these people honoring him with LSD." Some other Leary friends sent some of his ashes to outer space in 1997, but Sarandon kept some for this event. The chest holding Leary's ashes was placed below a photo of a nun with a cross between her legs. Next to the ashes was a photo of Leary and a sign reading "Gone fishin'."[3]

Susan has been interested in politics, having campaigned for John Edwards and Bernie Sanders. She was one of many actors in the documentary about how films depicted same-gender attraction and identified herself as being bisexual on the September 2022 *Tonight Show* starring Jimmy Fallon. She has spoken out that drug offenders are being unduly punished. She has advocated to end the death penalty, and was arrested June 28, 2018, for a sit-in protesting Donald Trump's migrant separation policy.

Sarandon has won many acting awards and was appointed UNICEF Goodwill Ambassador in 1999. She was one of eight women who carried the Olympic flag at the opening ceremony of the 2006 Olympic Winter Games in Turin, Italy. She received the Action Against Hunger Humanitarian Award in 2006, and donated fruit trees to the New York City Housing Authority's Jamaica Houses in 2018 in the borough of Queens, where she went to help plant the trees.

Notes

1. https://www.vogue.com/article/susan-sarandon-burning-man-timothy-leary
2. https://ew.com/articl/2015/09/11/susan-saran-timothy-leary-burning-man-video/
3. https://www.usatoday.com/story/life/2015/09/06/susan-sarandon-burning-man-timothy-leary-ashes-lsd/71801664/

Esther Williams

Esther Jane Williams (1921-2013) was an American competitive swimmer and actress. She set regional and national records in her late teens. She spent some months swimming alongside Olympic gold-medal winner and *Tarzan* star Johnny Weissmuller. Talent scouts noticed her, and she was soon appearing an "aguamusicals."

She appeared in movies and television specials and became a businesswoman before retiring from movies. She sold her name for bathing suits, properties, and pools. She first married Leonard Kovner from 1940-1944 who planned a career in medicine, actor/singer Ben Gage from 1945 to 1958 who squandered her money, Argentine actor/director Fernando Lamas from 1969 until his death in 1982, and actor Edward Bell whom she married in 1994.

Esther Williams wrote *The Million Dollar Mermaid: An Autobiography,* with D. Diehl, in 1999, published by Simon & Schuster. In the first chapter, she described how she came to use LSD, lysergic diethylamide, and what it did for her.

She described an interview with Larry King on *CNN* in November 1999, where she remarked that LSD was "instant psychiatry." In a clinical setting, she was able to relive an early repressed trauma while under the influence of LSD.

She wrote that she was a child during the economic depression of the 1930s and was the last of five children. She had grown up always feeling the need to please and care for her family. Although she was a popular movie star and leading actress in water musicals during the late 1940s and 1950s, she was in deep emotional pain over an immense feeing that she must achieve.

She was introduced in movies starring in 1942 *Andy Hardy's Double Life*. The swimming star kissed the young lad played by Mickey Rooney who went a little crazy in love with her.

> Rooney: You mean we can have a little cuddle tonight?"
> Williams: You mean the giraffe party?
> Rooney: Giraffe?
> William: Well, a giraffe has a long neck!

In the 1948 movie *On an Island with You,* she co-starred with Peter Lawford in one scene:

> Lawford: Put your arms around my neck.
> Williams: If I put my arms around your neck, I'd choke you!

While flying to Europe in 1959, she suffered a panic attack on the airplane. A kind flight attendant offered her an alcoholic drink. As she sat sipping it, she felt that something had to be done to lower the anxiety in her life. A divorce from her second husband had left her with IRS tax problems as her alcoholic husband had wasted almost ten million dollars through gambling and bad investments.

As she sipped her drink and thumbed through the September 1959, issue of *Look* magazine, she found an interview with Cary Grant. He related that he had, under a physician's supervision, taken LSD with remarkable effects. He explained that he did not truly know who he was. He said that the LSD experiences allowed him to make a rapid recovery from his emotional problems. He was quoted, "I am through with sadness. At last, I am close to happiness. After all those years, I'm rid of guilt complexes and fears."

The physician who treated him had said that LSD "empties the subconscious and intensifies emotion and memory a hundred times." Grant said that having money, beautiful women, and expensive houses had not brought happiness. He felt that it was important to know who you are.

She had known Grant for years but was not especially close to him. But she decided to call him after she landed. She wanted to know if he thought the psychedelic could be beneficial. He invited her to visit him at his office the next day. She was convinced after their conversation that she wanted to meet Dr. Hartman, so he helped her make an appointment.

She talked with the doctor about her wishes. He then took her to a darkened room where she took the prescribed dose of LSD and was told to lie down, not be afraid, close her eyes, and for two hours, let the psychedelic take effect. She was left alone during that time. She described the "trip" to be the most amazing journey of her life.

She first noticed that her body and resistance started to ease. Then she began to picture her father's face on the day that her beloved brother, aged sixteen, had died. She was only eight years old at the time. It seemed as if her father's face was like a plate that shattered into small pieces, and he became faceless. Her mother seemed to have no emotion at all.

She felt like she had returned to that devastating time when her good-looking brother with his acting talent had brought the family to California from Kansas, hoping that he would break into movies and had become the family hope. His death had left the parents without a reason to live, she thought.

Under the influence of the LSD, Esther began to wonder why her mother took her without the three older siblings to view the brother's dead body at the funeral home. Then she told Larry King, "I made a vow to replace him in my family, to heal my mother and father's devastation and be their 16-year-old-boy. I was too young at 8 to be that. So, I had to become sixteen." She said that she began to feel her brother's presence with her all the time. She realized the other children had various problems so they could not replace her brother. So, she felt she had to grow up overnight.

After Williams left Hartman's clinic, she spent that night with her family. She felt a very strong obligation to care for her parents in every way that she could. She retired early and looked at herself in the mirror after removing her makeup. It seemed to her as if she had become both a boy and a girl, taking her brother inside of her so that he became part of her. She felt that she finally understood who she was and what she had tried to do.

Esther Williams became famous for promoting swimming, making it attractive, and showing how it was good for health, exercise, and fun. She died of natural causes in 2013 at age 91.

CHAPTER SEVEN
Menninger's Clinic

Charles F. Menninger (1862-1953) was a physician who founded the Menninger Foundation with sons Karl and William. He was born in Indiana and completed his medical training at Chicago's Hanemann Medical College in 1889. He then moved to Topeka, Kansas, where a small medical school was being operated by the local medical community. He became a faculty member training on internal medicine and metabolic problems. Charles Menninger had been inspired by William W. Mayo who had come to America from England to found the Mayo Clinic in Rochester, Minnesota, with his two physician sons, William and Charles.[1]

In 1919, son Karl Menninger (1893-1990) completed medical training at Harvard Medical School in Boston and formed a partnership with his father, opening the Menninger Clinic in Topeka. His book, *The Human Mind* published in 1930, explained the science of psychiatry. Later, the clinic became the Menninger Foundation for the study and care of people suffering from mental illnesses.

Karl underwent psychoanalysis by Franz Alexander and Ruth Mack Brunswick, both of whom worked with Sigmund Freud. Karl went to Vienna with Alexander and met Freud in 1934. He invited Sigmund Freud to join the Menninger group but that never happened.[2]

Karl became good friends with Anna Freud and invited her to lecture and visit Topeka as a visiting scholar. She did so several times during the 1960s. He also helped form the Winter Veterans Administration Hospital in Topeka, which became the largest psychiatric training center in the world. In 1946, he founded the Menninger School of Psychiatry named in his honor.

He married Grace Gaines in 1916, and they had three children. After a divorce in 1941, he married Jeanette Lyle, and they adopted a daughter. He wrote other works including *The Crime of Punishment* believing that crime was preventable through psychiatric treatment, *The Vital Balance, Man Against Himself,* and *Love Against Hate.*

Karl met with former First Lady Eleanor Roosevelt in February 1959 and gave her a tour of the Topeka facilities. He was awarded the Presidential Medal of Freedom by Jimmy Carter in 1981.

William Menninger (1899-1966) graduated from Washburn University and went to Cornell University College of Medicine in New York state. Then he completed a two-year internship at Bellevue Hospital, and studied psychiatry at St. Elizabeth's Hospital in Washington, D.C. He married Catherine Wright in 1925 and they had three sons who each became active in Boy Scouts, reaching the rank of Eagle Scout.

William joined his father and brother in Topeka where he advocated the use of bibliotherapy in treating mental illness. He believed that self-help books such as those written by the Menninger family were helpful to patients. The Menningers thought that Sigmund Freud's belief that a psychologically sound person could work and love should be part of their treatment. Thus, they have beautiful gardens as did Anna Freud for people to grow various plants and foods. They also found work in the community for patients during their stay. Their staff showed great love and empathy toward all patients.

President John F. Kennedy met with Dr. William Menninger while sitting in his famous rocking chair in the Oval Office at the White House on February 9, 1962. Menninger explained that mental health care was at a turning point in history. He wanted President Kennedy to seize leadership on psychiatry which was the most neglected area of health causes. He said, "We want somebody of your stature who will stand up with us and be counted."[3] Little did Menninger know of Kennedy's addiction to Max Jacobson's amphetamine injections.

Menninger was appointed director of the Psychiatry Consultants Division in the Army at the outset of WWII. He chaired the committee that developed the first international classification of mental disorders in 1949. It preceded the first *Diagnostic and Statistical Manual of Mental Disorders* published in 1952. He attained the rank of brigadier general in the U.S. Army.[4]

Dr. Robert Wallerstein came to run the Menninger School of Psychiatry in 1949 and stayed for 17 years. He gave the farewell presentation at the closing of Menninger's on June 15, 2001. He began his talk by saying: "The first time I went, Akim Tamiroff was on the stage, and many other Hollywood stalwarts played in the Topeka Civic Theater in those days."[5]

The Menninger Clinic moved in June 2003 from Topeka, Kansas, to Houston, Texas. Old friend child psychoanalyst Roy Aruffo, M.D., was involved with the new setting up of Menninger's in Texas. As of May 2012, its new location is 12301 S. Main St., Houston, Texas. It offers adolescent and young adult programs, and psychiatric assessments.[6]

We will now look at some of the patients who were treated at the Menninger Clinic in Topeka, Kansas.

Note

1. http://www.kshs.org/archives/223942 and http://www.kshs.org/p/menninger-foundation-archives/13787 from the Kansas State Historical Society.
2. http://www.jstor.org/stable/26305298.
3. https://www.jstor.org/stable/j.ctt1ckpb9x.19
4. http://www.kshs.org/camp/units/view/224188 and https://books.google.com/books?id=8chrAAAAMAAJ
5. https://guilfordjouncals.com/doi/epdf/10.1521/bumc.66.4.320.23397
6. Robert S. Wallerstein, *Forty-two lives in treatment: a study of psychoanalysis and psychotherapy: the report of the Psychotherapy Research Project of the Menninger Foundation, 1954-1982,* New York: Other Press, 2000 *and American Academy of Child and Adolescent Psychiatry,* aacap.org/aacap/Life_Members/A_School_Experience.aspx

Brett Favre

Brett Favre was born in 1969 in Gulfport, Mississippi, and became a football quarterback who played in the National Football League for twenty seasons, primarily with the Green Bay Packers. He had 321 consecutive starts from 1992 to 2010, the most in league history. By the time of his retirement, he was the NFL leader in passing yards, passing touchdowns, quarterback wins, and holds the record for most interceptions. He was named Most Valuable Player three times and was inducted to the Pro Football Hall of Fame in 2016.

He used opiates and alcohol throughout his career until February 27, 1996, when he landed in the hospital for surgery to remove a bone spur and had a seizure. When he came to his senses, his doctors said he had a seizure and could have died. The physicians told him that his dependence on painkillers probably contributed to the seizure by withdrawal side effects.

Like so many professional athletes, they take an injection to keep playing after being hurt. His physicians had supplied the usual low doses of Vicodin. It made him want more and he tricked other players into giving him some of their supply. He had become addicted. He went to a rehabilitation facility as part of a 10-part treatment plan and was required to stop drinking for two years if he intended to continue playing with his football team.

However, in 1995, surgery and injuries caused him to use Vicodin heavily. He tried to hide his addiction, but his girlfriend and others found his hidden stashes and noted his insomnia. He was dehydrated, constipated, and irritable.

He struggled to keep his promises of quitting, but despite unannounced urine tests continued his substance abuse.

Finally, on a phone call to a friend, he said, "People look at me and say, 'I'd love to be that guy.' But if they knew what it took to be that guy, ... I'm entering a treatment center tomorrow. Would they love that?[1]

He had to report to the Menninger Clinic, or he would be fined some $900,000. He was terribly embarrassed in a press conference talking about it. But he entered on June 28, 1996, and completed a 46-day stay, where he was evaluated by a psychiatrist, attended group therapy, and overcame his addiction. He married his girlfriend and returned to football.[2]

Brett Favre did an interview with Dr. Phil. That was psychologist Phil McGraw with whom the author had some classes at North Texas State University (now called University of Texas) in a Dallas suburb. After McGraw did some work for Oprah Winfrey, she had him appear on her show and he now has a show helping people with problems.

Dr. Phil interviewed Favre in 2021, and Brett said about his drug abuse: "It sort of numbed the pain, but it also felt pretty good... It was two pills that gave me a buzz, and then it was four. At its peak, I was taking 16 Vicodins all at one time." He was able to get access to the additional pills from his teammates. He said, "You start learning how to manipulate the system, and you become very good at it."[3]

Brett was interviewed by Ross Bennelick for an article in *Sportskeeda* on November 8, 2022. He described his addiction problems saying that his first stay at Menninger's was for Vicodin addiction. His second was for alcohol addiction. He said:

I was in there 28 days, and it worked. When I got out, the toughest thing was the first three months, because I had to change my thought process. When I played golf before, I realized the only reason I wanted to play was to drink. After a while, instead of thinking, 'How many beers can we drink in 18 holes' I fell into a pattern of what could I do to get good at golf.[4]

Compared to other patients, Favre's were short stays. He probably complied with club rules for required length of treatment rather than psychiatrists' estimate of time needed for treatment.

On February 15, 2023, Bridget Hyland wrote an alert for *NJ.com Sports* that said: "The former quarterback is currently in the center of a scandal, and the man who wrote his biography has chimed in. Jeffer Pearlman, author of *Gunslinger: The Remarkable, Improbable, Iconic Life of Brett Favre,* published in 2016, has said "Don't buy my book, he's a bad guy." Why would the author say that?

Brett Favre was connected to a Mississippi welfare scandal involving the misappropriation of roughly $77 million in state funds. He is one of 47 defendants in a civil lawsuit against misspent welfare money. Three issues include (1) Favre being paid for appearances and speeches he did not attend, (2) his involvement with a drug company for which he was a spokesperson, and (3) tax records showing Favre funneled money from a charity supporting underserved and disabled children and breast cancer patients to the University of Southern Mississippi to build a new indoor football facility.[5]

This information certainly suggests that role models for children should be offered only after a lifetime of reputable behavior by a star can be shown. In addition, team doctors and coaches should think hard about giving athletes painkillers and sending them back to play without pain. They should also discuss use and abuse with all team members so friends can't be coerced into aiding each other with drugs.

Notes

1. https://vault.si.com/vault/1996/05/27/nhl-26norc-3d1-26zx-3d1430450275468
2. https://archiv.jsonline.com/sports/packers/45266162.html/
3. https://people.com/sports/brett-favre-opens-up-about-addiction-to-painkillers/
4. https://www.sportskeeda.com/nfl/nfl-brett-favre-recalls-drug-alcohol-addictions-canded-interview
5. https://www.cbssports.com/nfl/news/brett-favre-scandal-explained-ex-nfl-qb-is-accused-of-misusing-of-mississippi-state-welfare-funds/

Carl Panzram (American Serial Killer)

Carl Panzram (1891-1930) was born on a farm in Minnesota to East Prussian immigrants. When Carl was given writing materials by prison guard Henry Lesser, who believed in redemption, he wrote the story of his life on death row in 1929. He and six siblings were made to work on their farm after truancy laws were passed requiring children to go to school. When his parents were made to obey, they sent the children to school by day and had them work through the night. He wrote that he would get just two hours of sleep before he had to get up for school. His parents' punishments involved being chained and being starved.

He wrote that he was not liked by other children, and that his father abandoned the family when he was seven or eight. He was in juvenile court at age eight in 1899 for being drunk and disorderly. At age 11, he was arrested and jailed for being drunk and "incorrigible." His next arrest was for stealing some cake, apples, and a revolver from a neighbor's home.

In October 1903, his mother sent him to the Minnesota State Training School, and wrote that he was repeatedly beaten, tortured, and raped by staff members. He wrote that he hated that school so much he decided to burn it down and did so on July 7, 1905, without being caught.

In 1905, he was paroled from Red Wing Training School where he was sent for stealing money from his mothers' purse. At age 15, two weeks after a parole, he attempted to kill a Lutheran cleric with a gun. He ran away from home and lived on the road as a hobo, where he was often accosted and raped.

In 1906, he and fellow inmate James Benson escaped from Montana State Reform School and stole guns. They broke into stores, burned buildings and churches, and then went their separate ways. In 1907, Panzram enlisted in the U.S. Army. He refused to take orders from officers, was convicted of larceny for stealing supplies, and served time in Fort Leavenworth from 1908 to 1909. He was released with a dishonorable discharge.[1]

He wrote that he robbed and raped men. In 1911, he was using the alias of "Jefferson Davis" who had been the former president of the Confederate United States. He stole things while living as a logger in Oregon. He hid in a bordello where his wallet was stolen, he was infected with gonorrhea, and finally treated during another imprisonment. In 1915, he abetted another escapee who killed the warden of the Oregon State Penitentiary in Salem.

He escaped from prison in 1918 and sailed to Panama, Peru, Chile, London, Edinburgh, Paris, and Hamburg or so he said. He returned to the U.S. in 1920 and targeted the mansion of former President William Taft in New Haven, Connecticut, because of a sentence Taft gave him at Leavenworth. He stole jewelry, bonds, a handgun, and bought a yacht. He claimed to have killed sailors but was jailed for six months only on charges of burglary and possession of a loaded handgun.

He wrote that he caught a ship to South Africa and landed in Angola. He bought a girl of 11 or 12 whom he raped and returned her to family. He returned to the U.S. and raped and killed two boys. He committed more murders and was finally sentenced to 25 years to life at Leavenworth Federal Penitentiary. The foreman of the prison laundry harassed him, and he beat the man to death with an iron bar.

At his trial, the court requested Dr. Karl Menninger's assessment of the defendant's sanity. On the morning of April 15, 1930, in a small office inside the courthouse in Topeka, a meeting was arranged under court supervision. Panzram was brought into the room at 8:30 a.m. Thick, heavy chains were wrapped around his hands and arms and a stiff iron bar was attached to each ankle. He could walk only a half-step at a time with federal guards. He sat down in the chair and stared at Dr. Menninger.

"Good morning, Mr. Panzram," said Dr. Menninger. The prisoner turned his head away and said nothing. Then he said, "I want to be hanged and I don't want any interference by you or your filthy kind. I just know more about the world and the essential evil nature of man and don't play the hypocrite. I am proud of having killed off a few and regret that I didn't kill more!"

Dr. Menninger tried to get him to talk about his life, but he refused and became angrier and more impatient. "I am saying I am responsible, and I am guilty and the sooner they hang me, the better it will be and gladder I will be. So don't you go trying to interfere with it." The interview was terminated, and the prisoner was taken out of the room.

The next day, Dr. Menninger wrote a letter to Warden T. B. White. He asked to interview Panzram again. "For purely scientific purposes I should like to look into the case of Carl Panzram in a little more detail. His case was an extraordinary one as you know, and I am very interested in finding out what the earlier evidence of his mental instability were."

The warden refused further access. Having read the account of his life written by Panzram, Menninger blamed Panzram's adult hostility on the treatment he received as a child in the Minnesota state reform school at Red Wing. He later wrote about the case in his 1938 book *Man Against Himself,* where he used the pen name of "John Smith" and identified Panzram as prisoner No. 31614, which was the number on the plaque of his prison grave.

Menninger said, "The injustices perpetrated upon a child arouse in him unendurable reactions of retaliation which the child must repress and postpone but which sooner or later come in in some form or another, that the wages of sin is death, that murder breeds suicide, that to kill is only to be killed."[2]

Robert Stroud, the so-called Birdman of Alcatraz, who was in prison until he died in 1963 later wrote that Panzram was restless the night before his execution. "All night long that last night he walked the floor of his cell, singing a pornographic little song that he had composed himself."

Panzram said the death sentence was a relief and he resisted attempts to have a stay of execution. He said, "I look forward to a seat in the electric chair or dance at the end of a rope just like some folks do for their wedding night."

He was then convicted and sentenced to death. He refused any appeals of his sentence. Death penalty opponents and human rights activists tried to intervene, but he wrote: "The only thanks you and your kind will ever get from me for your efforts on my behalf is that I wish you all had one neck and that I had my hands on it... I have no desire whatever to reform myself. My only desire is to reform people who try to reform me, and I believe that the only way to reform people is to kill 'em!"

On death row, officer Henry Philip Lesser gave him money to buy cigarettes. The prisoner was so surprised that they began to chat. The officer gave him writing materials and he wrote the story of his life. He began his journal stating: "In my lifetime I have murdered 21 human beings, I have committed thousands of burglaries, robberies, larcenies, arsons, and last but not least I have committed sodomy on more than 1,000 male human beings. For all these things I am not in the least bit sorry. I have no conscience so that does not worry me."[3]

On May 30, 1930, Panzram wrote President Herbert Hoover over concern about a possible change in sentencing. He said he was "perfectly satisfied with my trial and the sentence. I do not want another trial... I absolutely refuse to accept either a pardon or a commutation should either or the other be offered to me."

On the morning of September 5, 1930, Panzram was taken to the scaffold by two U.S. Marshals and faced a crowd of officials, journalists, and guards. He climbed the 13 steps to the platform and stood erect. As the Marshal attempted to place a black hood over his head, he spat in his face. When asked for any last words, he said, "Yes. Hurry it up, you Hoosier bastard. I could kill a dozen men while you're screwing around!"

The Marshals stepped back, and the trap doors sprung open with a crash. He dropped five and a half feet down, his large body jerking, and swung from side to side in silence.

Guard Henry Lesser who gave him the materials to write his autobiography worked long and hard to find someone to publish the memoir. It finally was published by Thomas Gaddis and Joe Long. Thomas Gaddis had written the 1955 book *Birdman of Alcatraz* which was made into a movie with Burt Lancaster playing Robert Stroud.

Killer: A Journal of Murder was published in 1970 and became the basis for a 1995 movie entitled *Killer: A Journal of Murder*, with James Woods playing Panzram. John Bedford Lloyd played Dr. Karl Menninger in the film.

Notes

1. https://military-history.com/wiki/Carl_Panzram
2. https://www.psychologytoday.com/us/blog/shadow-boxing/202007/the-meanest-man-who-ever-lived
3. https://oac.cdlib.org/findaid/ark:/130030/c82j6cf9/admin/

Akim Tamiroff

Akim Mikhailovich Tamiroff (1899-1972) was born in Tbilisi, Georgia, in the Russian Empire. His father worked in the oil fields in Baku on the Caspian Sea. He was of Armenian ethnicity and trained at the Moscow Art Theatre drama school in 1920. He arrived in the United States on a tour with a troupe of actors in 1923. He decided to stay because he fell in love with a Russian lady in America. He became an actor with a very thick Russian accent. He was told never to remove that accent since it was used when he portrayed foreigners in movies.

At first, he worked in New York and did Russian nightclub acts with his wife, Russian-born Tamara Shayne, whom he married in 1933. He also worked for entertainer Nikita Balieff in his famous Bat Cabaret. Balieff was a Russian Armenian who had a touring theater in Paris and then New York. He hired dancers, singers, and actors. Then Tamiroff opened his own make-up studio where young Katherine Hepburn was one of his students. They would both star together in the 1944 *Dragon Seed* movie with Walter Huston.

He appeared on Broadway in several events including *Miracle at Verdun* in 1931, where he played Roubeau. He toured America with Al Jolson in *The Wonder Bar*. Jolson's fame in movies began with the *Jazz Singer* in 1927 and he made movies for about five years. He then returned to Broadway and toured with the Wonder Bar group including Tamiroff from 1931-1934.

Akim was in several movie roles without credit until 1935 when he co-starred in *The Lives of a Bengal Lancer* with Gary Cooper, Franchot Tone and C. Aubrey Smith.

He next starred in the 1936 movie, *The General Died at Dawn* with Gary Cooper and Madeleine Carroll. He played the General and was nominated for Best Supporting Actor. He said that Gary Cooper brought him good luck.[1]

He appeared in the 1937 *High, Wide, and Handsome* with Irene Dunne and Randolph Scott. He played an excellent role winning much acclaim in the 1938 *Dangerous to Know* with Anna May Wong, Anthony Quinn, and Lloyd Nolan. He was nominated for Best Supporting Actor in *For Whom the Bell Tolls* starring Ingrid Bergman and Gary Cooper. Here is some dialogue between Tamiroff and Katina Paxinou.

> Tamiroff: Here I command!
> Paxinou: Here I command. Haven't you heard them? Here no one commands but me now.
> Tamiroff: I should shoot you and the foreigner both.
> Paxinou: Try it and see what happens. Listen to me, drunkard! You understand now who commands?
> Tamiroff: Why, I command!
> Paxinou: No, Listen! Take the wax from your ears. Listen well. I command.
> Tamiroff: All right. All right. You command.

Orson Welles chose him to play in *Touch of Evil, Mr. Aarkadin, The Trial,* and the unfinished *Don Quixote*. In the latter, he was to play Sancho Panza and went with Welles to Europe but was never paid for his work and time on that picture. In the Tamiroff papers which can be accessed on the Internet, a rough picture of Tamiroff done by Orson Welles in pen and ink or crayon can be seen.[2]

Tamiroff also starred in *The Great McGinty, Ocean's Eleven, Topkapi* and many other movies in well-paid roles.

In the 1940 movie *The Great McGinty* with Brian Donlevy, Akim played the role of a man who used malaprops (a wrong word which is like the right word) for comic effect. He played the role so well that he inspired the cartoon character Boris Badenov on *The Rocky and Bullwinkle Show* of cartoon characters. The creators of the show credited Tamiroff's explosive temper and accent from *The Great McGinty* as their model for the character. Swedish actress Greta Garbo in *Ninotchka* inspired the Natasha character on that show.[3]

In 1943, he created a mutual aid society for needy Russian actors in Hollywood. He remained in that post for nine years and became needy himself during that time. He helped men such as Russian actor Michael Chekhov, nephew of playwright Anton Chekhov, and student of Konstantin Stanislavski. Michael played the role of the Freudian analyst in Alfred Hitchcock's 1945 *Spellbound*. In fact, Tamiroff was extremely helpful to Chekhov, holding classes and soirees where Chekhov could meet actors such as Anthony Quinn, Lloyd Bridges, and Mala Powers. Akim would occasionally tell others how he was cast in many movies as Mexican or Spanish and got little credit in his early movie years.[4]

Akim Tamiroff was a patient at the Menninger Clinic from 1949 to 1951, off and on. Like so many stars, he went through psychoanalytic psychotherapy and possibly analysis as well. He struggled with his career but enjoyed acting at the local theatre during his time in Topeka. He returned to making movies in 1951 until he died of cancer in 1972. One of his closest friends was another Russian born actor, Mischa Auer.

Notes

1. vintoz.com/blogs/vintage-movie-resources/Mischa-auer-and-akim-tamiroff-by-way-of- russia
2. https://www.wellesnet.com/don-quixote-orson-welles-secret/
3. https://www.avclub.com/low-rated-and-barely-animated-rocky-bullwinkle-becam-1798239117 and https://content.time.com/time/magazine/article/0,9171,2028066-2,00.html
4. https://russianlandmarks.wordpress.com/2015/09/30/akim-tamiroff-home-beverly-hills-ca/

Gene Tierney

Gene Eliza Tierney (1920-1991) was born to a successful insurance broker and his wife, a former physical education instructor. Gene was raised well and spent two years in Switzerland in a sort of finishing school where she became fluent in French. She returned to the United States and while visiting Warner Brothers studios with her family, Director Anatole Litvak spotted her and told her she should become an actress.

Her parents had groomed her to be a debutante and she made her society debut in 1938 at age 17. Bored with that life, she told her parents she wanted to study acting and her father paid for her to act in a Greenwich Village acting studio in New York.

Her first Broadway role was in 1938, and she received acclaim from critics in both 1938 and 1939. Her father set up a corporation to fund and promote her acting career. Columbia Pictures signed her to a six-month contract in 1939. She met Howard Hughes, who wanted to seduce her. She was not impressed but they became lifelong friends.

She began her movie career in 1940 with *The Return of Frank James* with Henry Fonda. She played in John Ford's 1941 *Tobacco Road* and the title role in *Belle Starr* with Randolph Scott in 1941. She met Oleg Cassini whom she married in 1941 and divorced in 1952. Her parents were so upset about their relationship that they eloped. Later, her father tried to take away some 25% of her movie earnings but was unable to do so.

Oleg was a stylish dress designer, and grandson of a Russian-Italian count who was the czar's minister of China and ambassador to the U.S.[1] He had a younger brother,

Igor, who wrote under the byline Cholly Knickerbocker and was the Hearst newspaper chain's gossip columnist for New York. Gene Tierney wore the clothing Oleg designed in her movies. He would later become famous as the designer of First Lady Jacqueline Kennedy's clothing line. Gene was in the 1943 comedy *Heaven Can Wait*.

In June 1943, Gene Tierney became pregnant and took a break from movies but appeared at a WWII USO party at the Hollywood Canteen. She shortly became ill with German measles (rubella) while she was pregnant. Tierney got through her week or two of illness and recovered. However, her baby girl, Daria, was born deaf and severely retarded.

A female Marine ran into her on a tennis court a year or so later, and laughingly confided that she snuck out of quarantine with German measles to meet her idol Tierney. She asked if Gene caught the illness. Gene simply walked away, as this explained her child's problems. However, she and Oleg Cassini had another daughter who was born without problems.

Howard Hughes is mentioned several times in this book. He was the son of Howard Robard Hughes, a Houston man who founded the Hughes Tool Company. The father invented a two-cone rotary drill bit that penetrated hard rock at ten times the speed of any former bit and that revolutionized oil well drilling. He died when son Howard was eighteen, so Howard Hughes Jr. became the sole owner of the Hughes Tool Company.

Young Hughes married from 1925 to 1929 "football queen" Ella Botts Rice, niece of William Marsh Rice for whom Rice University is named. They moved to California so Howard could produce movies, but he also flew airplanes setting records, ran businesses, and met many interesting people such as Cary Grant, Randolph Scott, Errol Flynn, Carole Lombard, Billie Dove, Ida Lupino, Bette Davis, Ava Gardner, Olivia de Havilland, Katharine Hepburn, Fay Wray, Ginger Rogers, and Gene Tierney. Hughes second wife from 1957 to 1971 was actress Jean Peters.[2]

Hughes had severe pain from a plane crash in 1945 and his physician, Dr. Norman Crane, gave him codeine and valium, which Hughes abused, and he died from kidney damage after years of over-using those drugs.[3]

The medical bills for Gene Tierney's daughter Daria were so high that her old friend Howard Hughes paid for her to have the best possible care in the beginning. Gene always remembered his kindness.

In 1944, her big movie hit was *Laura*. That movie was perhaps the most memorable of Tierney's era, as a notable film noir about a woman who was seemingly murdered but reappeared later. By this time, she had begun to have episodes of depression followed by overactive mania and sleeplessness. She had started smoking to deepen her voice and was becoming a very heavy smoker, which would finally result in her death from emphysema.

Her role in the 1945 *Leave Her to Heaven* with Cornel Wilde brought a nomination for Best Actress. She played the role of a woman who was self-possessed and cared nothing for anyone but herself. She was next filming the 1946 *Dragonwyck*. A dreamy position as governess with a rich relative played by Vincent Price becomes evil and sinister. Here is some dialogue with Walter Huston:

Tierney: But there's everything here you could possibly want.

Huston: Everything is what no man should ever want.

While that film was being made, WWII veteran John F. Kennedy came on the set. She wrote about him in her 1978 autobiography *Self-Portrait*. She met him again at the house of skater Sonja Henie. They danced and she fell for his Irish charm. They had in common her underdeveloped daughter Daria and his sister Rosemary who was born retarded. They dated for nearly a year and once went to a French restaurant in New York City where they heard Edith Piaf sing. Tierney translated the French for John.

She asked the young man questions and listened with curious smiles, for he had a way of talking that was so odd and amusing. He was quite different from anyone she had ever known or heard before. He had such big ideas.

She and Oleg Cassini had separated, and Kennedy was her new love interest. Gene took him to meet her mother, and she fed him milk and cookies in the kitchen. Her family did not see any future in her dating a Catholic since they were Episcopalians, and she was about to be divorced. Oleg, who would become Jacqueline Kennedy's favorite designer, knew the Kennedy family. He and her mother warned her that Jack could not marry a divorced woman. Then, one day Kennedy told her of his political ambitions and that he could not marry her and still be seen as a proper Catholic running for office.[4]

In 1946, Tierney made *The Razor's Edge*, 1947 *The Ghost and Mrs. Muir*, and 1950 *Where the Sidewalk Ends*. In 1950, she went to London to film another noir picture, *Night and the City*. Jules Dassin directed that movie, and it was his last Hollywood film since the witch hunt for communists became so serious that he never returned to the United States. The moody movie was extremely well-done, featuring Richard Widmark, Gene Tierney, Herbert Lom, and Frances Sullivan.

In 1952, she and Cassini divorced but remained friends until her death. She was filming *Personal Affair* and began a romance with Pince Aly Khan, and they became engaged in 1952. Aly was a Pakastani diplomat who was going through a divorce from Rita Hayworth. He had known Orson Welles in his youth, and by interesting coincidence, both he and Orson had been married to Rita. Aly's father, Aga Kahn III, was upset with his son's romances, and did not want his son to be involved with another actress. Hayworth and Aly were married in 1949, had daughter Yasman, and their 1953 divorce was becoming a custody battle.

Aly explained the problem to Gene and dropped his engagement. She had transferred a huge ring Aly gave her to her right hand as if it were an engagement but moved it back to her left hand. By 1953, Tierney was suffering with problems of concentration. She dropped out of *Mogambo* and was replaced by Grace Kelly.

When 1955 *The Left Hand of God* with Humphrey Bogart and Gene Tierney was being filmed, Tierney was mentally ill. Since Bogart's sister, Pat, had mental illness, and Bogie had paid for her illness, he recognized the symptoms. He fed Tierney her lines since she had trouble memorizing them, and he strongly urged her to get help.

She went to the Institute of Living in Hartford, Connecticut. Movie silent star Clara Bow, the "It Girl" was given shock therapy there for schizophrenia in 1949. Gene Tierney was given 26 shock treatments but finally fled from the hospital.

Electroconvulsive therapy (ECT) is where a generalized seizure (without muscular convulsions) is electrically induced to alleviate unmanageable mental disorders such as major depression, mania, and catatonia. Typically, 70 to

120 volts are applied externally to the patient's head for about six seconds. The most common adverse effects are confusion and transient memory loss. The usual course of ECT involves multiple administrations, typically given 2-3 times per week until the patient no longer has symptoms. Gene later became an opponent of shock treatment therapy saying it had destroyed much of her memory.

She felt suicidal in 1957 and went up to the 14th floor of her mother's apartment and stood on a ledge outside the window. Police were summoned and talked her down. She was finally admitted to Menninger's Clinic and was in treatment with psychotherapy for some two years. Part of her therapy was to begin to act and live like a normal person. So, she took a job as a clothing salesgirl in Topeka by day and returned to the clinic each night.[5]

She said that her problem was "my lack of understanding of what I could cope with and what I couldn't cope with. I learned that to carry on while you're broken is not the answer. I tried to work harder and harder, thinking that work would cure everything. All it did was make things worse."[6]

One day, the press learned that actress Gene Tierney was working as a salesperson near Menninger's and printed a story that made her very upset. It affected how people saw her and there was a stigma about being a psychiatric patient in those days. She had to work through that as well as her other problems. She finally believed that she had conquered her problems and was discharged. She wrote in her autobiography that she felt like a "lab rat" in other treatment centers, but Menninger's had helped her to feel normal again.[7]

She returned to Hollywood after six years of treatment at three mental hospitals and many electric shock treatments and made three more films: 1962 *Advise and Consent,* 1964 *Toys in the Attic,* and 1964 *The Pleasure Seekers.* She made only a few appearances on television after that.

She met oil tycoon W. Howard Lee who had been married twice, actress Hedy Lamarr being his second wife, and they married in 1960 in Aspen, Colorado. Lee and Tierney lived together in a quiet and fulfilling marriage in Houston, Texas, until his death in 1981. She died at age 70 in 1991, of emphysema.

Her daughter Daria spent most of her life at the ELWYN institution for specially disabled people in Vineland, New Jersey. Her obituary was written by her sister, Christina "Tina" Cassini:

> My loving sister Daria Cassini ended her journey on September 11, 2010, just prior to her 67th birthday, October 15. She will always be remembered in the thoughts and prayers of our mother's and father's families (Gene Tierney Lee and Oleg Cassini) and in the hearts of my four children and six grandchildren and those who cared for her.

Christina Cassini died in poverty in Paris in 2015. She had ovarian cancer and was the divorced mother of four grown children. She was bequeathed a million dollars by Oleg Cassini as the daughter of Gene Tierney. However, Cassini's widow never allowed her to have that money, despite knowing of Christina's cancer. Thus, not only did Gene Tierney have a tragic life, so did her normal daughter, who had buried her incapacitated sister five years earlier.[8]

Notes

1. https://www.vanityfair.com/news/2010/09/oleg-cassini-201009
2. https://spartacus-educational.com/JFKhughesH.htm and bill37mccurdy.com/2010/08/13/hughes-new-howards-first-marriage/
3. https://www.nytimes.com/1077/06/26/archives/hughes-death-laid-to-massive-drug-use-illegally-obtained-medicines.html
4. https://www.irishcentral.com/roots/gene-tierney-john-f-kennedy
5. https://people.com/archive/gene-tierney-began-her-trip-back-from-madness-on-a-ledge-14-floors-above-the-street-vol-11-no-18/
6. https://content-time.com/time/subscriber/article/0,33009,821205,00.html
7. https://www.nytimes.com/1991/11/08/moview/gene-tierney-70-star-of-laura-and-leave-her-to-heaven-dies.html)
8. https://pagesix.com/2015/04/06/oleg-casinnis-daughter-dies-in-poverty/

Robert Walker

Robert Walker (1918-1951) was born to parents who divorced when he was a child. His aunt, then president of Bonwit Teller, encouraged his interest in acting and paid his tuition at the American Academy of Dramatic Arts in New York City in 1937. There, he met Phylis Isley whose stage name later was Jennifer Jones. They married in Tulsa, Oklahoma, in 1939.

Walker was in some small unbilled parts in movies. Their son, Robert Walker Jr. (1940-2019) became an actor in later years. Their other son, Michael Walker (1941-2007) was an actor who appeared in movies and on TV series.

Robert and Phylis Walker worked in Hollywood where Walker had limited success. Phylis auditioned for producer David O. Selznick in 1941 and was chosen for a movie contract. Robert starred in 1943 *Bataan,* 1943 *Madame Curie,* 1944 *See Here, Private Hargrove,* 1944 *Thirty Seconds Over Tokyo,* and 1945 *Since You Went Away.*

Wife, Jennifer Jones, starred in a 15-chapter serial, and in 1943, won the Academy Award for Best Actress in *The Song of Bernadette*. During the filming of that movie, she began an affair with Selznick. The Walkers separated in 1943, but she co-starred with him in *Since You Went Away*. They divorced in 1945 and she married Selznick in 1949 until his death in 1965. She then married philanthropist Norton Simon in 1971 until his death in 1993.

Walker was devastated by their divorce and co-starring with her tortured him. He tried to move on and was in 1945 *The Clock* with Judy Garland, and 1945 *Her Highness and the Bellboy* with Hedy Lamarr and June Allyson. He was in the musical 1946 *Till the Clouds Roll By* playing Jerome

Kern, and 1947 *The Sea of Grass* with Spencer Tracy and Katharine Hepburn.

In 1948, while making *One Touch of Venus* with Ava Garner, he married Barbara Ford, the daughter of director John Ford. The marriage lasted only five weeks. John was furious about Barbara's union with Walker.

Robert Walker was drinking heavily and was required by the motion picture studio to spend time at the Menninger Clinic in Topeka, Kansas, where he was treated for a psychiatric disorder. He spent some six months there and underwent psychoanalysis. He returned, interacted with his two sons, and began dating. He continued his psychotherapy with Viennese psychiatrist Frederick Hacker, M.D. Hacker was recommended by Louis B. Mayer because he had earlier treated Judy Garland.[1]

Walker was cast in Alfred Hitchcock's 1951 *Strangers on a Train* where he astutely played a charming psychopathic killer. He was killed in the movie's final scenes on a merry-go-round. He then went into production for his next movie where he was thrilled to play with the famous Helen Hays. That movie was the 1952 *My Son John*. Walker died before production finished so parts of his death scene in *Strangers on a Train* were spliced into the death scene in *My Son John*.

Unaware of the tragedy that would later befall Robert Walker, Hitchcock had thrown in some amusing dialog, as was his want to do. In one scene, Walker is talking with his mother played by Marion Lome:

Lome: Well, I do hope you've forgotten about that silly little plan of yours.
Walker: Which one?
Lome: About blowing up the White House.

Walker: Oh, Ma. I was only fooling. Besides, what would the President say?

Lome: You're a naughty boy, Bruno.

That excellent movie won wide acclaim. He may have been very unhappy despite the new movie with Hays. On August 28, 1951, Robert Walker's housekeeper found him in an emotional state. It is unknown whether he had been drinking or not. She called his psychiatrist, Dr. Hacker. The psychiatrist rushed over and administered amobarbital for sedation. Walker lost consciousness and stopped breathing. He was pronounced dead at age 32. No autopsy was requested but it was considered possible that Robert Walker had drunk heavily that day and the amobarbital-alcohol combination killed him.

After his death, ex-wife Jennifer Jones who married millionaire Norton Simon invested in mental health causes. She was quoted in an article called "Team for Mental Health" by Phyllis Battelle, in the Lancaster, Ohio, *Eagle-Gazette* article of June 26, 1980: "I have been in psychotherapy since I was 24, and still am...I have attempted suicide three times when I was in deep despair."

She added that her daughter by Selznick, Mary Jennifer, had plunged to her death at age 22 from a hotel roof. Her husband, Norton Simon, had been in psychotherapy since the early 1950s. Jennifer and Norton both brought their psychoanalysts to meet their expected partners before marriage. All went well and the couple married and created the Jennifer Jones Simon Foundation for Mental Health and Education, which offered workshops on mental health problems research, and treatment. Jennifer said: "I hope we can re-educate the world to see there's no more need for stigma in mental illness than there is for cancer."

Much information is available about Robert Walker and Jennifer Jones in the book *Star Crossed: The Story of Robert Walker and Jennifer Jones* by Beverly Linet, 1985, New York: G. P. Putnam's Sons.

Note

1. https://www.robertwalkertribute.com/1949-51pacificpalisades.html

CHAPTER EIGHT
Selecting a Doctor

We have seen both good and bad doctors and some of their results with patients. We all see doctors and there may be important things to keep in mind when we see a new doctor for the first time. After all, we can always change our minds and choose someone else if we are not pleased by that first contact. What should we look for in the doctor who will take care of our life?

Each person has a different set of standards. A friend of mine (Gary B.) gave me this description of what he would like to see in a doctor's office:

> I want my doctor to be an effective advocate for me. It all starts in their office. Do they answer the phone politely, with concern and a true interest in helping do what is being asked? Are the Assistants, PA's and others who interact with patients informed, well-trained, and understand their limitations? Are appointment times kept? Do they approach their assignments knowing that they represent the doctor, so must deal with all issues in a sincere and caring way.
>
> Is the doctor up to speed on the latest and greatest information, symptoms, remedies, surgical techniques, prescription medications, etc. Is he/she willing to

commit the time and energy to test, diagnose and recommend actions that will address the issues causing the appointment?

Lastly, is there a follow-up contact from the doctor or his office to insure that all is progressing as necessary to resolve the problem? That contact may also include a survey to be submitted by the patient or their advocate rating the experience of dealing with the doctor and his staff.

Let us see studies that have been made by the American Medical Association about what most patients want from their doctors:

Eye contact is important instead of a doctor who is looking at his computer screen asking questions. Patients want a partnership and need to be consulted about their condition, treatment, and possible progress from their consultation. They want enough time to explain things and have the doctor explain his diagnosis and treatment plan. Patients want a doctor who looks healthy, who takes care of himself or herself, and has an organized office as if care is taken to prevent germs and disorder. A doctor should display an attitude of liking people and wanting to help them.

1. Transparency: Your doctor does not have to know everything, but he/she should share as much as possible. Uncertainty is okay. If a doctor has committed an error of any kind, it should be shared with assurance that the doctor is trying to fix the error. In addition, the success rate and risks of procedures should be shared with patients.

2. Patients want a doctor who listens as they describe health issues and symptoms, respects the patient's opinion, and asks questions to understand the cause of their illness. Too much of a time rush can never be beneficial to anyone involved.
3. A patient will trust a doctor who is an active listener and who understands that they are asking personal questions that will be kept confidential.
4. Patients want face-to-face interaction without financial incentives getting in the way. Over-treatment with tests and major costs is not equal to better care.
5. Respect the needs of a patient such as feeling cold when a blanket would help, water for someone who is thirsty, waiting 45 minutes and then spending only 5 minutes with them during the appointment.
6. Communication must be effective so doctors must be ready to explain things in a way the patient can understand.
7. Some patients require more time than others so that they can understand things more completely.
8. A doctor should show empathy by learning about the daily routine and lifestyle preferences of a patient, as well as discussing possible side effects of medications.
9. Access for sick patients is necessary. They should not have to wait for weeks on lab results and make numerous calls to receive them. Electronic health records help with access in many cases. Appointments must be made as quickly as possible with patients who are ailing or in jeopardy.
10. Clear instructions about tests, treatment, and possible results and written directions improve communication between doctors and patients and reduce phone calls.

11. If patients must consent to certain tests or treatment, talk it through until they understand the purpose and implications of a test or treatment. Patients have rights and must participate in their healthcare rather than being inactive in the care plan.

The philosophy of doctors and how they work has changed over the years. In the 21st century, our vision of the world has gradually developed through science. Science forces us to take responsibility for the welfare of ourselves, our species, and our planet. Health care is being reshaped by evidence-based medicine. Treatments are now being tested to display evidence about their good, bad, and indifferent results.

Scientific discoveries set the pace of our lives. We cannot all be scientists, but we trust our physicians to be scientific enough to help us survive and thrive. We have become a people who are fitted with a sense of sympathy and the ability to reflect upon our own predicament. We have been raised and educated to think up and share new ideas. Our physicians are among the most educated in the world about health.

We live in a world that has increased life and health in most industrialized countries, but the United States has fallen behind 65 other countries, yet it has the most wealth. Why? The darker sides of human nature have infested American life with guns, drugs, and risky behaviors.

Despite those behaviors, we are continually pushing ourselves forward with ingenuity, sympathy, and good institutions. Patients have as large a role in human health as physicians who are carefully trained to understand health and how the body works. We must be carefully trained in how to live our lives. Let us look to good people and good principles to help us.

www.ingramcontent.com/pod-product-compliance
Lightning Source LLC
LaVergne TN
LVHW091533060526
838200LV00036B/594